MW00902576

Death In The Afternoon

How To Control Drinking In The 21st Century

RAEGAN BAKER

Published by Raegan Baker

https://www.raeganbaker.com

Cover Design by Jacquelyn Loerop and Erica McCary,
GoodLight Creative

Printed by Createspace

Manufactured in the United States of America

Death In The Afternoon:
How To Control Drinking In The 21st Century

Copyright © 2019 by Raegan Baker

All rights reserved. No part of this book may be
reproduced in any form or by any electronic or
mechanical means, including information storage and
retrieval systems or transmitted in any form or by any
means – electronic, mechanical, photography, recording,
scanning or other – except for brief quotations in the
critical reviews or articles, without permission in writing
from the publisher.

Raegan Baker

Death In The Afternoon:
How To Control Drinking In The 21st Century

First Publishing 2019

ISBN: 9781096224815

Table Of Contents

Dedicated to Hannah, Katie, Marlee, Meg and Shelby

And to everyone who wishes to break free from being dependent on alcohol. You have no idea how strong you are. It is possible.

Acknowledgements

As I reached the completion of this book and prepared to send the manuscript to my editor, I realized that I had not yet come up with a title. After much thought, I decided *Death In The Afternoon: How To Control Drinking In The 21st Century* was an appropriate, meaningful one. The drink 'Death in the Afternoon' was invented by famed novelist Ernest Hemmingway. It is a cocktail made up of absinthe and champagne, and shares a name with Hemingway's book *Death In The Afternoon*, published in 1932. Having always idolized successful authors who came before me, I found this title fitting for this reason, and for the fact that Hemmingway himself has gone down in history not just for his popular literary works, but also for his alcohol abuse.

I am fortunate that alcohol dependency did not steal years from my life. All things considered, my time relying on drinking to "help me cope with life" was relatively brief. However, in that time I managed to do a lot of damage in regard to work, relationships and everyday life in general. After about six months of alcohol controlling my life, I enrolled in a treatment center for three months. I then followed up with eight months of additional therapy in which my counselor, an Eye Movement Desensitization and Reprocessing (EMDR) specialist, and I worked on the traumas that had caused me to "pick up" in the first place. After our sessions came to a close, I spent countless hours attending Alcoholics Anonymous (AA) meetings.

While all of this helped me to a certain degree, the true turning point in which I decided to give up drinking 100% was when I started to read the life changing book *This Naked Mind* by Annie Grace. Prior to this, I always had it in the back of my mind that I would go back to "normal" drinking, consuming alcohol at happy hours and social gatherings like I had before it took over my life. Annie Grace changed that thought completely. I can honestly thank her and the wonderful book she produced for likely saving my life. This is no exaggeration. As a writer, I find it fitting that it was a book that intervened and prevented me from the possibility of total self-destruction. I am honored that she has asked me to share my story on her podcast in the coming months. I view her as an amazing mentor. She has done so much for those who suffer from alcohol abuse. If I can make half the impact that she has, then I will have done my job.

Introduction

I am going to do something that will perhaps shock most of you. If you are an alcohol "virgin," I am not going to ask you to never drink. I am not going to talk down to you for wondering what alcohol tastes like. I will not berate you for your curiosity. Inquisitiveness about the unknown is natural if you are young and entering new stages of life. And if you have consumed beer, liquor or wine before, I am not going to ask you to stop, or to never bring any of those liquids towards your lips again.

What I am going to do is ask you to really take in the words you are about to read in this book, and to fully grasp exactly WHAT alcohol is, how it is portrayed in our society, how to recognize the difference between the facts and myths regarding this substance and how it has interfered with the lives of people from all walks of life.

If you had told me a year ago that I would one day write this book, I would have looked at you as if YOU were drunk. However here I am now, a completely different person with a completely different outlook on alcohol than just 12 short months ago.

In order to understand why I state that I am no longer the same individual with the same view of drinking as I once was, you need to truly get to know me. I know many of you reading this now will be able to relate to me and my background.

My childhood was an ideal one. I was born and raised in the picturesque city of Richmond, Virginia, a place of natural beauty that is steeped in American History. I was blessed with a loving family, many friends and my closest childhood companion was my loyal, loving dog Sugar, a medium-sized collie mix. I attended a private school from kindergarten until the sixth grade. Halloween was (and still is) my favorite holiday. Thanksgiving, Christmas and Easter meant many gifts, enormous feasts and making amazing memories with my cousins and siblings, memories that I will always cherish. And my summers involved countless days at the local pool while the nights were spent catching lightening bugs with the neighborhood kids. It was a childhood I wouldn't trade for the world. And as you may have already guessed, alcohol played absolutely no role in my life as I was growing up. I was completely shielded from people who drank. I never witnessed that side of life during my first twelve years on this earth.

By junior high my family had moved from the city to the suburbs and I happily switched over to a public school. I was excited about the change. Most of my friends from my elementary days were beginning to move away, so I looked forward to meeting new people. Best of all my cousin, who was like a fourth sibling to me, would be making the switch over to the same public school.

Starting at a new school, one with a student population of about 1,000, meant I was suddenly exposed to kids my age that came from much harsher backgrounds than my own. That said, I remained largely naïve about the cruel realities of the world, including addiction.

It wasn't until I was 13 when I was finally exposed to alcohol for the first time. It was a crisp, winter day. School was closed due to snow. Three neighborhood girls knocked on my front door and asked if I wanted to join them for a walk. I quickly grabbed my coat, hat and gloves and dashed outside. Once we approached a field on the edge of some woods, we stopped walking. They pulled out wine and beer, enough for all four of us. I cracked open my can and took my very first sip of Miller Lite. I honestly don't remember much other than I thought it tasted absolutely disgusting, and I was amazed to see one of my friends chug her can as if it were a Diet Coke.

That was the first time I ever had alcohol, and the experience was so unappealing that I didn't take another sip until college. You read that right, I didn't drink again until college. I went through my entire high school career without taking in a drop of alcohol. And it wasn't like I was some outcast student who didn't partake in the traditional high school experience. In fact, the opposite was true.

In many ways I was like millions of other American teens at the time. My weekends were spent with friends attending our high school football games, shopping at the nearby mall to grab the latest fashion trend, hanging out at the local movie theater and spending countless hours on the phone discussing the latest

Friends episode (this was the 90's after all). Alcohol never played a role in my life during those years. Classmates and friends would sneak it on occasion (some more than others), but I was never pressured into drinking. I chose not to, and no one seemed to mind either way, so it just wasn't an issue for me.

I graduated from high school in the spring of 1999 with an excellent GPA, even winning an award for my hard work. That fall I began my college career in Virginia Beach, Virginia, a tourist city with plenty to do along the shores of the Atlantic Ocean. However, just like high school, drinking did not play a major role in my life.

I honestly think I drank a total of ten times during that entire four-year period. I attended parties across campus and at friends' apartments, but I rarely consumed any alcohol then, and I certainly didn't experiment with any illegal drugs. I would bring a Diet Coke to parties, attending to simply enjoy time with friends and meet new people. I wasn't against drinking at the time, and I didn't mind that many of my friends would stumble back to their dorm rooms intoxicated (it was their choice after all), I just never had the desire to drink.

When college ended and I had earned my B.A. in Communications, I immediately applied, and was accepted to, a graduate school that was also located in Virginia Beach. These would turn out to be some of the best years of my life. I entered the program at age 23 and immediately formed amazing new friendships while maintaining most of my old ones from college as well. During this amazing two-year period, I won a scholarship to study abroad at Oxford University in England for one summer. I traveled with friends to New York City, Mexico and Russia (twice). I also started to work on my first book that would eventually be published and sold out due to popular demand. Most importantly, I completed my degree, earning an M.A. in Public Policy.

It was also during this time that my drinking finally started to increase, however not to the point that it interfered with life. Sunday through Thursday were dedicated strictly to school and work (when I wasn't in class, I was working at my university's library). However, I allowed myself to let loose and relax on my Fridays and Saturdays. I would spend the days shopping, going to lunch with my roommate at our favorite Indian restaurant and laying out at the beach. However, what I most looked forward to on these days off from school and work were the nights. I had a very close circle of friends and every Friday and Saturday evening were spent playing volleyball followed by enjoying each other's company at someone's apartment or house, drinking our favorite alcoholic beverages while playing card games, building bonfires and just relishing our time together as carefree, young 20-somethings.

It was during this time that I "discovered" mixed drinks. Prior to that, I had only tasted beer and wine coolers, not enjoying either. However, when I was introduced to rum and coke, vodka and cranberry juice and a host of other combined beverages, I started to develop a taste for alcohol. Still though, it never once interfered with school or work, so I never thought I was doing anything wrong. Not to mention alcohol is legal, which sent me the message that everything was okay. Little did my naïve brain know I was building a tolerance to a very toxic poison.

By the time I had completed my graduate program, I was all of 25 and ready to take on the world. I entered politics and started working in Washington, D.C. My office had a perfect view of the city. Yet I was still so young and so naïve. I had stars in my eyes every time I walked by the U.S. Capitol or the White House. It was the equivalent of a young adult wanting to go into acting and arriving in Hollywood. That's the best description I have of my feelings as I went to work every day in the nation's capital.

It was at this time that my weekend drinking with friends slowly started to turn into weeknight drinking with co-workers at happy hours or political events. Yet, it still wasn't an issue. It didn't interfere with my job during the day, and it wasn't out of the norm for everyone I worked with (whether in the office or around the political scene in the city) to wine and dine at the strike of 5:00 pm and last for three to four hours. I never felt particularly pressured to drink with them, I did it because I thought that's just what a person in politics did after office hours. I was following their example, and since alcohol is a legal substance, I never imagined that these seemingly innocent after work drinking episodes would eventually lead down a destructive path.

Fast forward five years. By this time, I was in my early 30's and I had moved out to California to attempt my PhD. While the degree ended up eluding me, I spent three years in the Golden State, enjoying a different lifestyle on the West Coast. I lived in San Diego, basking in year-round sunshine that often lead to many outdoor activities. I also traveled to other parts of the state, including San Francisco and Yosemite National Park. Those were three memorable years that I will always look back on and smile at the memories. Yet without realizing it, my alcohol consumption continued to slowly grow like it had when I first entered the working world in Washington, D.C., however now I was increasing the amounts I took in.

It started evolving even more due to the first roommate I had when I moved out west. For the first time in my life, I had more free time to spend meeting and dating new and interesting men, ones different than any I had been with before back east. It was exciting, but nerve racking at the same time. My roommate suggested I have a drink before each date, claiming that the alcohol would allow me to relax and that it would take the edge off, making me less nervous. Sadly, I took her advice, and soon I was drinking not only to relax, but to also fall asleep easier at night. It wasn't long before I was relying on alcohol for almost every situation, considering it a "go to" thing if I ever needed it for any emotion that I felt. If I was happy, I drank. If I was sad, I drank. If I was celebrating an accomplishment, I drank. It was becoming a part of my daily routine. Yet it still didn't interfere with work, family, friends or life in general. I didn't realize that I had become a "functioning alcoholic."

I had no idea what was in store for me when I said goodbye to California after three years and headed back east. I planned to return to the political world, however one day back in Washington D.C., I ended up being attacked by a person I was supposed to trust. This occurred almost two years ago, and my drinking went from being something that occurred mostly at night to something I did no matter the time. It could be 6:00 in the morning, and I would easily down a can of beer or several shots of vodka. It didn't matter what I poured down my throat so long as I passed out. That was my goal, to fade out of consciousness and to not think, not feel.

After about eight months of this horrific way of life, I entered a treatment program in another state that would include daily AA meetings. While treatment and AA can certainly help some people out there, I needed something else. I think it's wonderful that many people gain their sobriety back this way, however it doesn't work for everyone. I continued to drink, and it still was a destructive force in my life. I started at another treatment center immediately after my time at the first one ended. I began Eye Movement Desensitization and Reprocessing therapy (EMDR) that would address my Post Traumatic Stress Disorder concerning the attack, as well as other issues from my 30 plus years of life that needed to be attended to. I completed eight months of much needed therapy, but I still had the desire to drink. It would be sporadic days here and there, but the point is it still happened. In moments when trauma became overwhelming, I still viewed alcohol as a "friend" that could help me get through it.

That all changed when I saw an online advertisement for the book *This Naked Mind* by Annie Grace. It claimed to have a different approach to alcohol, a more scientific one. I ordered the book, started to read it, and as they say, the rest is history.

This Naked Mind explained to me just what alcohol truly is and how our society leads us to believe countless myths about drinking, myths that have over time come to be viewed as facts. Grace made a statement that really clicked with me; that willpower is often not enough to fight addiction. Remember, alcohol kills thousands of people all over the world every year. We need to realize how alcohol impacts our brains and blurs the line between fact and fiction. We need to stop viewing it as something positive and realize the truth; that it is not only a drug, but the deadliest drug out there. Just because it is legal in most parts of the world does not change this fact.

And that is what this book is about. As I stated at the beginning of this introduction, I am not going to ask you to never drink. Nor will I lecture you if you already have, or if you already consume alcohol on a regular basis. Again, I'm only asking you to read the words in this book and truly take it all in. When you finish this book, I want you to have a complete understanding on what alcohol is, how it is portrayed in society and the facts and myths surrounding it. Most importantly I want you to become fully aware that anyone can fall victim to abusing this very powerful liquid.

Many of you may believe that you are not prone to becoming dependent on this poison because alcoholism does not run in your family. I am living proof that is one of the many myths concerning alcohol. You read about my upbringing, how alcohol played no role in my childhood. No one in my immediate family had a problem with addiction. I never drank in high school and I rarely consumed it in college. But even I wasn't safe from its clutches. It nearly took me down, seemingly out of the blue, when I hit my mid-30's. If it can happen to me, it can happen to anyone. No one is safe from this toxic liquid. Absolutely no one.

So, I only ask of you to read this book with an open mind, and to come away with the full knowledge of what alcohol is and how it can destroy a person's life and everything that he or she have worked years to accomplish.

Thank you for taking the time to absorb the words that you will read on the following pages.

I truly thank you.

CHAPTER 1:

The Myths That Surround Drinking

In my early 30's I had moved out to California and began using alcohol as a "crutch." My roommate had suggested I take shots before I went on first dates to "take the edge off" so I could "relax" when meeting these intriguing men for the first time. I listened to her, and hence a snowball effect happened in which I started to rely on alcohol to deal with every emotion: anxiety, excitement, happiness, grief. You name it. I had come to believe I absolutely NEEDED alcohol in my life, no matter the situation. And that is what this first chapter is about: the myth of NEEDING alcohol.

Our society has glamorized drinking. Think about how many times you have seen an advertisement on television that shows a good-looking guy cracking open a can of beer surrounded by beautiful women on a sunny beach lined with swaying palm trees. The advertisement is sending viewers the message that attractive people drink, therefore in order to be physically appealing you must have a drink in your hand. It also causes a person to think that he or she can somehow land a beautiful date if alcohol is involved.

How about the sitcom in which one of the main characters just broke up with her boyfriend of five years? They had plans to marry, start a family and live happily ever after in a beautiful home located in an affluent town. Her friends gather around to comfort her, with one handing her a cold beer. Suddenly the heartbroken young woman looks up from her tear-soaked tissues and smiles as she takes a sip from the bottle. She dries her eyes and her sadness magically starts to evaporate.

What about the commercial that shows a loving, middle-age couple fulfilling their lifelong dream of touring through the breathtaking towns across Italy? At one point they are seated in an elegant restaurant, while sharing a bottle of expensive red wine. The commercial is portraying that this wine is needed to top off their memorable evening, that the night wouldn't be complete without alcohol being involved. What the commercial doesn't show is the intoxicated 20-something college student, stumbling around in a dark alley just a few blocks away and completely at the mercy of someone who would want to take advantage of her.

We have been programmed by our society into thinking that alcohol is needed in our lives. We have been led to believe it is something that will help us land an attractive partner, help us better enjoy our long-anticipated vacation, that it will help ease our emotional pain when we are heartbroken and depressed.

Nothing could be further from the truth. I repeat: Nothing could be further from the truth.

I will take each of the examples above in which society has programmed us into believing drinking is the answer to every problem/situation and prove how that belief is a dangerous fallacy.

Let's look at the young man drinking a beer on the beautiful beach with lovely, adoring women swarming around him. Do you really think that in real life this guy, no matter how good looking he is, would draw in attractive young woman in a tropical setting just because he is downing a drink? Of course not. You are intelligent enough to know that the very idea is ludicrous. However, without realizing it, your subconscious mind is tucking this advertisement away, and without realizing it you begin to associate drinking beer with being physically appealing and having the ability to attract good-looking people into your corner.

What about the sitcom centered around the heartbroken young woman who was just shattered after her plans of marrying the love of her life fell through? Remember how her caring friends handed her a drink, and suddenly she was able to smile again? In reality, alcohol is a depressant. It does not help a devastated individual feel better. In fact, the opposite is true.

Alcohol has a sedative effect on the brain. Many people believe a couple of beers or a glass of wine can relieve stress, when the truth is alcohol can put you at an increased risk of despair. Alcohol is a depressant that can cause your problems to seem worse than they are, and it can make you feel even more miserable than before you had a drink.

People who abuse alcohol have the highest rates of depression. That includes those who drink to "feel better." Studies have shown that 30 to 50 percent of people who abuse alcohol this way suffer depressive symptoms at any given time. Drinking does not lift their spirits; it only makes their feelings of anguish worse.

Neuroscientist George F. Koob, PhD., is an internationally-recognized expert on alcohol and stress. He found that drinking reduces our levels of serotonin and dopamine. These are natural, feel-good chemicals that keep us peaceful and optimistic. Therefore, we become more depressed, not more jovial, when alcohol is consumed.

"The worst thing you can do if you're depressed is to drink," claims Dr. Howard Samuels, CEO/Founder of The Hills Treatment Center located in Los Angeles, California. "A lot of people are drinking because they're depressed and then that makes their depression 10 times worse."

Even if a person is not feeling down when he or she begins a night of drinking, it does not guarantee that the person won't eventually become irritable, anxious and depressed as the alcohol consumption increases. Remember that drinking has a negative effect on serotonin and dopamine, those feel-good chemicals in the brain. As a result, one does not feel better as a night of drinking wears on, they feel worse.

Now let's examine the commercial involving the older couple on their dream vacation through Italy. It suggests that drinking is needed to heighten their already good time, as if the wine is necessary. That without it their trip just won't be as memorable.

Of course, we know that is complete nonsense. Drinking will not magically make their vacation better. Yet that message seeps into our subconscious, and we begin to believe we need alcohol in order to make an already good time even better when that is simply not the case.

How about alcohol and bravery? Have you ever heard of the "liquid courage" myth? It is the widely held belief that alcohol is necessary to give someone a fearless "boost" when they are experiencing feelings of dread, intimidation, or even nervousness. Remember, I fell for this extremely absurd, yet commonly believed fallacy, when my roommate in California suggested I take a few shots of vodka before a first date in order to "take the edge off." Sadly, I did just that, and from there on I started to associate alcohol with being a cure for almost every emotion, just like I had been programmed to believe by Hollywood when I was growing up.

Annie Grace authored her groundbreaking book on controlling alcohol titled *This Naked Mind*. She devoted an entire chapter to the topic of liquid courage. Grace wrote about the fact that she, like countless other people, becomes nervous before she must give a public speech. She had also once fallen for the myth that alcohol can make a person more confident, therefore she would have a few drinks before speaking in front of others. She eventually realized that alcohol did not boost her confidence but rather chipped away at it.

Grace stated that while sober, even when nervous, she would prepare and rehearse a speech. She would be in complete control of the planning, and as a result she would be 100% prepared by the time she stepped in front of a crowd of people. However, if she added alcohol to the mix just before giving her much prepared speech, she neglected rehearsing. Not surprisingly, her speeches got worse as she continually added drinking before them to the mix.

In a 2016 article Grace penned for the *New York Daily News*, she explained the connection between alcohol and the nerves. "Alcohol and anxiety are actually the best of friends – they go hand in hand. The very act of drinking can increase your anxiety and leave you feeling worse once it wears off. While alcohol might initially relax you because it is a sedative, it changes levels of serotonin and other transmitters in your brain. Your anxiety levels can be off the charts after drinking," she wrote.

What about people who state that they drink "for the taste?" Is alcohol, something people instinctively spit out if they first attempt to drink it as small children, something that is truly appealing to our taste buds? Grace devoted a chapter of *This Naked Mind* to this topic as well.

When I took my first sip of alcohol at age 13, the taste was so terrible I had to force myself to swallow it so I wouldn't look like an amateur in front of my more experienced friends. There is no question that is most people's experience the first time they consume this toxic liquid – the desire to spit it right back out. So why do we keep drinking it, and why do we eventually come to think we enjoy it?

Have you ever heard the phrase "you need to acquire the taste?" Someone once said that to me when I remarked on how I found Red Bull disgusting after I tried it for the first time. People make the same comment when it comes to alcohol. I eventually built up a taste for Red Bull, and sadly I did the same for alcohol. Just like the energy drink so many rely on first thing in the morning to get moving for the day, alcohol becomes a liquid we build up a tolerance for and start to believe we can't live without.

What about people who claim drinking beer, liquor or wine makes them happy? We have already touched on how alcohol is a depressant, that science has proven it does not help to lift someone's mood. Yet people have been brainwashed into believing that drinking brings them joy. Maybe you are one of those people.

Alcohol is responsible for so much misery in the world. It causes the successful CEO to eventually neglect his job responsibilities, causing him to lose his once admired position. It allows a once loving mother to ignore her children's needs, leaving them starved for food, love and attention because she is more focused on finding a way to get her next bottle of wine. It has destroyed friendships and entire families. In fact, 70% of alcohol-related violence takes place in the home. Yet people (maybe even you) claim it makes them happy. Alcohol, which has caused thousands to be raped and murdered, which has led once prominent people into homelessness, which has allowed parents to abandon their innocent children, is the root for so much pain and self-destruction. Yet thousands out there believe that they have, by some miracle, dodged this bullet. Alcohol has been the downfall of so many lives for hundreds upon hundreds of years, yet they are somehow special enough to be immune from its devastation.

Alcohol does not provide happiness. It causes misery. No one is immune from falling prey to its dark clutches. Anyone who drinks runs the risk of eventually going down a dark, destructive path.

Then there is the myth that alcohol is needed in order to maintain a social life. As teenagers and young adults, this belief is prevalent. But think back to when you were a small child at a birthday party or play date. Did you need alcohol in order to enjoy a fun-filled day of Red Rover, cake and whacking the pinata? Did you need to guzzle down a few cans of beers to enjoy playing Barbie Dolls with your best friend? Of course not! But alcohol has become so ingrained in our society that people have forgotten as they get older that there was once a time when they had fun without drinking.

You may fear that you will have to give up social events if you decide not to drink. That is understandable. There was a time when I couldn't have imagined going to a happy hour and not ordering a rum and Diet Coke. However now I just order a Diet Coke. I am aware of the dangers alcohol brings, and that is enough for me to enjoy my social engagements without downing any liquor. Your friends may get defensive at first. In fact, without realizing it, they may start to defend their reasons for drinking when they see you have decided to pass up the alcohol. However, eventually they may realize that you are enjoying your time despite not feeling the need to get tipsy, and it will become apparent that alcohol is not what is responsible for you having fun and happily engaging with others.

Many people believe that being prone to alcoholism is inherited through our genes, that if a parent is an alcoholic, then his or her offspring is more at risk to become one, too. Studies have shown that children of parents who suffered from alcoholism are approximately 4 times more likely to have problems with alcohol.

The well-known Recovery Village is a network of facilities that offers comprehensive treatment for substance abuse disorders. The organization's website states, "There have been many studies showing there are genetic factors influencing alcoholism, specifically as it relates to children of suffering alcoholics. These studies show children from families with alcohol abusers are twice as likely as the general population to suffer from alcohol-related issues. However, there isn't a specific alcoholic gene that appears in a person's DNA. Instead there are behavioral genes that influence a predisposition to alcoholism, including mental illnesses. Also, different combinations of genes influence the level of alcohol consumption."

In other words, genes may certainly factor into a person developing a dependency on alcohol, however, they are in no way the only factor. In fact, there are many, many risk factors that play a role in the development of an alcohol addiction. These risk factors interact differently in every individual, leading to alcohol use disorders in some people but not in others. Some of these risk factors are psychological, social and environmental.

Countless people are under the assumption that if alcoholism does not run in his or her family, then he or she is immune from going down the devastating path of alcoholism. I am living proof that is simply not true. No one in my immediate family had a problem with abusing alcohol or any other kind of drug. (And yes, alcohol is indeed a drug. We will dive into this fact later in the book).

According to the American Addition Centers' website, "When people are exposed to large amounts of an addictive substance over an extended period of time, it is likely that this substance abuse will rewire the user's brain to crave the substance. Even without a genetic component present, a person can still inherit a predisposition to alcohol use disorder due to the culture they grow up in."

I believe that this is, to an extent, what happened to me. While I did not grow up watching family members drink, I did witness plenty of alcohol consumption on television and in the movies. Like the examples provided at the beginning of the chapter, I saw alcohol portrayed by the entertainment world as a "gift" of sorts, that it could enhance our happiness, cure our loneliness and basically aid us in any emotion – negative or positive – that we were experiencing. Even though I did not drink in high school, and very rarely in college, the belief that alcohol was the "be all, cure all" had already been firmly planted in my subconscious.

We are told by society that alcohol is our "friend," that we must drink it in order to feel better, enhance our good time, be the life of the party. These are all myths, and dangerous ones at that. It is not our friend, it is our very destructive enemy. We have been led to believe that if addiction does not run in our family, we will never fall victim to abusing alcohol or any other drug. That too, is a myth.

Alcohol does not discriminate. Everyone is at risk.

CHAPTER 2:

The Countless Victims

Let's revisit the commercial showing the couple sipping their wine on their glamourous trip through a southern European country. What it doesn't show is what often occurs in real life. Just a few short blocks from where a husband and wife drink their desired alcoholic beverage, the chances are great that an intoxicated college female is being hurt, or worse, by an individual who is taking advantage of her intoxicated state. This happens far too often, and alcohol advertisements certainly don't show this dark side of drinking. Just one (of literally thousands of examples) is that of an 18-year-old Virginia student named Hannah, whose tragic story made headlines across the world.

Let's get something straight from the get-go: Hannah was not an unintelligent young woman. She was extremely bright, as the university she attended and excelled in is a very prestigious school. However, alcohol impaired her thinking, and as a result, she violently lost her life.

In September of 2014, the college sophomore had attended a party in which drinking was involved. Sometime after midnight, she left the party to attend a second one. However, due to the amount of alcohol she had consumed, she became disoriented near a shopping center. Surveillance cameras captured her stumbling as she ran through the college town streets. She sent texts to her friends, informing them she was lost. Then, she was never heard from again.

Hannah was abducted in the pre-dawn hours by a 32-year-old criminal. Her remains were found one month later in a field not far from where she disappeared. It was later determined that the man who took her life was a serial killer, responsible for the death of another Virginia college student five years earlier.

Today, years after Hannah's brutal murder, her friends and classmates have graduated from college and entered the working world. Some have gone on to begin their desired careers, others have traveled the world, while many have married and started their own families. Yet Hannah remains eternally 18. She is forever frozen in time on those surveillance videos. A promising life cut short after a night of drinking.

While Hannah's slaying was the work of a serial killer with an extensive criminal background, alcohol has led otherwise law-abiding citizens to commit murder. Countless times it has caused people to go into a random fit of rage and kill their family members and friends. One very tragic example of this is the story of Marlee, who in 2018 was celebrating her birthday when her intoxicated husband shot her and two of their friends to death.

That night, Marlee, her husband and several friends had gathered for a small get-together to ring in Marlee's 27th year. At some point she hid her husband's car keys, likely realizing he had consumed too much alcohol to operate a vehicle. Outraged, her husband grabbed a .40 caliber pistol, slapped a cigarette out of his wife's hand, then fatally shot her. He then turned his attention to two of their friends after they tried to intervene, killing them as well. Three people were dead all because one person had too much to drink.

According to a sheriff who became part of the investigation after the murders, no other drugs were involved, just alcohol. He stated, "These were good friends having a nice time together." However, the husband became belligerent and resulted to murder all because his wife was trying to prevent him from driving drunk.

Sadly, Hannah and Marlee are only two examples of how alcohol has played a role in a horrific loss of life. Of course, not all deaths that involve drinking are the result of murder. As you already know, drunk driving is responsible for innocent people losing their precious lives on a daily basis. According to the National Institute of Alcohol Abuse and Alcoholism, nearly 10,000 are killed by drunk driving every year in the United States alone. That's one person every 48 minutes. Countless people who are sober and driving responsibly have their lives stolen by others who made the decision to operate a vehicle while intoxicated.

Among those who lose their lives are innocent mothers who will never see their children grow up, and many of them are not even in a vehicle when their lives were snuffed out. One infamous example of this involves another Virginia woman, one by the name of Meg. Her story made international headlines after she was struck by an intoxicated driver.

In January of 2014 she was on an early morning jog with her husband after seeing her three children off to school. At some point a car came barreling down the road. Meg and her husband scrambled to get out of its path, but the man behind the wheel struck the 34-year-old woman, killing her.

It was later learned that the intoxicated driver was a respected doctor. Yet despite the fact he was a well-educated person with a positive reputation, he still made the decision to drive after having too many drinks the night before, ending Meg's life. It was determined that his blood alcohol level was .11, well above the legal limit in Virginia, which is .08.

He was sentenced to ten years in prison for killing Meg, with six years suspended. Therefore, he will be locked behind bars for four long years, yet his victim will never see another sunrise, she will never celebrate another Christmas or watch her children grow up and start families of their own.

Meg's daughter, who was five at the time of her mother's senseless death, will never have a mother to turn to when she enters her teen years. She will never be able to confide her deepest secrets to her mother, ask for her for advice, or cry on her mother's shoulder when she experiences her first high school crush. This little girl will only have a grave to visit at a time in her life when she needs her mother the most. And perhaps the most heartbreaking fact of all is her memories of her loving mother will be vague at best, for she was only in preschool when her mom was taken away so senselessly.

Another innocent victim of drunk driving is the horrific case of seven-year-old Katie, a sweet-faced girl from New York. Katie was among a host of family and friends who attended her aunt's wedding on a warm, joyful summer evening in 2005.

That day, little Katie was spotted on the beach with her younger sister, happily tossing rocks into the Long Island Sound. As the guests happily dined on fine food and wedding cake, no one could have imagined it would be the last full day of Katie's life. When the festive event began to wind down near midnight, Katie, her sister, parents and grandparents eventually climbed into a limousine to journey back home. At some point along the ride, a car barreling down the wrong side of the highway at 70 miles an hour crashed into the limousine, shattering it to pieces.

The limousine driver was killed instantly, while Katie's family members were sprawled across the vehicle severely injured. Katie's mother, Jennifer, looked around the devastation. Blood was splattered throughout the limousine and broken glass littered the road. But where was Katie? Jennifer managed to climb out of the crushed vehicle and started to search for her little girl, who had been seated close to her and buckled before the crash. Then, Jennifer made a gruesome discovery. Katie had been decapitated by her seatbelt.

Perhaps in a state of horrific shock, the mother picked up and cradled her daughter's head, refusing to hand it over to paramedics who arrived on the scene. "I got numb. I thought I was going to collapse. All she was holding was this kid's head," a police officer later claimed. "I looked into the back of the limousine and I saw Katie's remains. She was wearing this dress and I just started shaking."

What if Katie had been a member of your family? Can you imagine laughing with your grandfather, mother or younger sibling one minute and then picking up their severed head the next, the rest of their body still strapped in a seatbelt? You would have to live with that horrific imagine for the rest of your life. It would never leave your thoughts, no matter how long you live.

The man who smashed into Katie's limousine had consumed around 14 drinks earlier that evening. By the time he got behind the wheel, his blood alcohol level was three times the legal limit. He was given an extremely harsh sentence which many, especially little Katie's family, believe he fully deserves. The man was convicted on two counts of second-degree murder and related charges. He's serving his 18-year sentence at a correctional center in New York.

Now, in a sense, his life is over, too. Because he made the decision to drive while intoxicated, which resulted in the death of an innocent child, he will not be released from prison for nearly two decades. He will go almost 20 years without enjoying the simple pleasures of life; pleasures like decorating a Christmas tree, enjoying a warm day with friends at a local beach or just being able to watch whatever movie he feels in the mood for. Simple pleasures you take for granted. Instead, his life will consist of a cold cell, little contact with his loved ones and three basic meals a day.

Of course, little Katie has it worse. She will never get the chance to grow up, experience high school, graduate from college, marry, or have children of her own. These two lives are forever destroyed because of one person's decision to drive while intoxicated.

Murder and drunk driving are certainly not the only causes of death when people consume too much alcohol. I'm sure you have already heard of alcohol poisoning, the severe elevation of the BAC (Blood Alcohol Content) which may lead to coma and death, often resulting from consumption of large amounts of alcohol. Death from alcohol poisoning is not rare; thousands fall victim to it every year. Many times, alcohol poisoning is the result of binge drinking, which is often defined as four or more drinks during a two-hour period for women and five or more for men. About 90% of the alcohol consumed by youth under the age of 21 in the United States is in the form of binge drinks. This is a frightening fact, given how many young people binge drink every year.

I could produce an entire book on real life stories of teenagers and college students (not to mention older adults) who have lost their lives to a night of binge drinking. However, I will use just one example, which is the heartbreaking story of a California girl named Shelby. The petite brunette was a gifted volleyball player who also ran cross country. She performed well academically and came from a loving, protective family. Her mother was a former police woman, yet Shelby succeeded in getting away with underage drinking, which eventually took her life.

Just before Christmas in 2008, Shelby attended a house party where alcohol was available to all the underage guests. Shelby's drink of choice was vodka, and her goal that night was to down 15 shots of it. "She wasn't this wild party girl. Shelby partied like most of us did. She didn't stand out as a troubled or moody kid. She was curious about alcohol — curious about how much she could drink until she passed out, just like many other teens.

You just drink until you're out, and then you sleep it off," one of Shelby's friends claimed.

Shelby started to consume the shots around 1:00 in the morning. She started to send off text messages to friends halfway through her goal, informing them of what she was trying to achieve. People responded, trying to convince her to stop. One friend even told Shelby she would get sick. One hour after she began her quest to swallow 15 shots, a friend led a heavily intoxicated Shelby into a bathroom and propped her up against the toilet in case she would need to vomit. She then left Shelby alone in the bathroom, rejoining the rest of the party until everyone finally decided to go to sleep.

The next morning, a friend was met with a horrific sight when she entered the bathroom Shelby had been left alone in hours earlier. The high school athlete was motionless. Her head hung over the edge of the toilet bowl, her lip split from having slammed against the porcelain from violent heaving. Her face was streaked with blood. EMTS were quick to arrive on the scene, but it was too late. The vivacious young girl who wanted to impress others by taking 15 shots of vodka was pronounced dead at 9:40 that morning.

While teenagers and young adults are prone to binge drinking, which often leads to death, the fact remains that every age group is at risk of this. I am an example of this. I did not drink a single sip of alcohol in high school and rarely in college. I became a weekend drinker in my mid-20's when I was in graduate school, and then I enjoyed a couple of beverages during the weekday happy hours when I became a young professional working in

Washington D.C. However, binge drinking was never a goal, nor a real issue, during those years. It wasn't until my late 30's when I almost died from consuming too much alcohol – once even landing in the hospital with a .370 blood alcohol content. You read that right, a .370. Many people are dead by the time they reach a .4. I am lucky to be alive.

It was one week during the fall. Thanksgiving was over, and the Christmas season was about to begin. I was extremely depressed. It would be the first Christmas without my beloved grandmother, who had passed away just two months earlier. I was also dealing with other family – and life – issues, and it had gotten overwhelming. Remember what I mentioned before about alcohol being a depressant? For several days I had downed countless shots of vodka to "erase" my pain; yet knowing deep down that I was only making it worse.

One night I sent an alarming text to my friend, which I would have never done if I had been sober. Thankfully she took over the situation and called an Uber to take me to the hospital. After a short wait in the in lobby, I heard her feet racing to my side. She had also once fallen victim to the horrors of drinking, and at that point she was eight years sober. She knew what I was going through.

After I was checked in and in a waiting room, I passed out. A little while later I woke up and vomited all over the floor. Of course, I was horribly intoxicated, so I wasn't fazed by the disgusting bile that I had just splattered everywhere. Instead I laid back down and a nurse had to come in and clean it up. My blood was drawn, and I was informed of that frightening number: .370.

I spent three days in the hospital recovering. If my friend had not called an Uber and met me at the hospital, there is a very, very good chance I would not be typing these words today. That's when I realized that if I didn't stop drinking, alcohol would eventually claim my life.

Billboards, commercials and sitcoms portray alcohol in a positive light. They show this toxic liquid as a necessary tool to aid the depressed, help the uptight relax and add enjoyment to an otherwise difficult day. Billboards don't display photos of people like Hannah, a promising young woman stolen from the world by a serial killer after what was supposed to be an "innocent" night of college drinking. Pro-alcohol commercials don't advertise horrific cases like Katie, who was decapitated by a drunk driver. And sitcoms certainly don't portray a main character like Shelby, dying alone on a cold bathroom floor after trying to accomplish swallowing a certain number of shots.

CHAPTER 3:

Alcohol Is A Drug

We hear it all the time. People say drugs AND alcohol. It has become such a prevalent phrase that without realizing it, we do not view alcohol in the same category as cocaine, heroin or methamphetamines. Since alcohol is legal in all 50 states and throughout most of the world, we don't consider it to be nearly as dangerous as the street drugs we read about online or hear about on televised news reports. If we are an American over the age of 21, we think to ourselves, "It's not like I'm breaking the law by purchasing this six pack of beer, what's the harm? It's not like I'm buying crack on the street corner from some dealer."

What we don't realize is that we are drinking a very toxic poison. Yes, that is exactly what alcohol is. It alters our mind, changes our personalities, damages our bodies, destroys our families, ruins our friendships and steals our money. Drinking it is no different than snorting a line of cocaine or shooting up a syringe full of heroin. In fact, in many, many ways alcohol is even worse. Just because it is legal throughout the world does not change this fact.

About six months after my drinking had spun completely out of control, I decided to enter a three-month treatment program in Florida. Now you must understand that when I entered this program, I still had the attitude that alcohol was not the same as the deadly street drugs we have all come to know. While I was fully aware that drinking can lead to drunk driving crashes, and that heavy alcohol use could damage a person's liver overtime, that was all I really knew when it came to the dangers of drinking too much. I was completely naïve about the true horrors that alcohol abuse inflicts on people. I thought to myself, "Yes, I need to learn how to control my drinking, but come on, I'm not like my roommate, the 15-year heroin addict." I thought I was "better" than most of my peers because my drug of choice was legal. I didn't realize that I was quickly going down the same destructive path as my roommate, who shot heroin into her veins, the guy who favored crystal meth and the 20-something who craved cocaine. My choice of drug wasn't against the law, so I wasn't in the same kind of danger they were in. Or so I thought.

Imagine my absolute shock when, after my arrival to the treatment center, I discovered cold, horrifying facts about alcohol that I had been completely unaware of before. Prior to my time in Florida, I did not know that alcohol withdrawal runs the risk of killing a person when he or she decides to stop drinking, yet coming off heroin does not. In that sense alone, alcohol is deadlier. I was also unaware of delirium tremens, the frightening side effect of alcohol withdrawal that does not run the risk of occurring in people who stop using cocaine, heroin or methamphetamines. And I certainly did not know that heavy alcohol use can damage a person's brain cells much like street drugs do, even if the drinker gives up the toxic liquid for good.

The reason I didn't know about these terrifying facts isn't because I was stupid. It was because I lacked the knowledge about the many, many dangers of alcohol abuse due to the fact that our society rarely touches on them. Every day thousands of people go online to keep up to date on the events that are making the news. Every day we read about the current horrors of the opioid crisis; how it is destroying countless lives by the minute. However, the horrors of delirium tremens, going into a coma from drinking too much, or dying from alcohol withdrawal is not making the headlines like the dangers of heroin use is. That is frightening because alcohol is now killing more people than opioids.

According to a November 2018 *USA Today* article, alcohol abuse in the United States is on the rise, and "it's an increase that has been obscured by the opioid epidemic. But alcohol kills more people each year than overdoses – through cancer, liver cirrhosis, pancreatitis and suicide, among other ways." The Institute for Health Metrics and Evaluation at the University of Washington reported that from 2007 to 2017, the number of deaths attributable to alcohol increased 35 percent. Death by drinking is an epidemic, and it isn't capturing the world's attention like the opioid crisis is.

Why is this? It is likely, in part, because of the fact that alcohol is legal. Every week talk shows air episodes about mothers who preach the dangers of heroin after their children overdose and die because the drug they took was actually the deadly fentanyl passed off as heroin. Every week we read stories online about once-promising high school athletes falling victim to the opioid epidemic and losing their college scholarships. Every day people log onto social media sites and learn about someone they grew up with who died from injecting these street drugs.

However, we are not bombarded with daily reminders that alcohol is killing even more people every day than opioids are. We are not being told that this legal drug that we are walking into the grocery store and purchasing runs a higher risk of killing us than the illegal drug we are trying to score in the dark alley behind the grocery store.

Alcohol is the world's most acceptable drug. However, if you ask the average person walking down the street to list all the deadly drugs he or she can think of, that person will likely leave it off the list entirely. "There continues to be a reluctance to accept that alcohol is an addictive substance because it's legal, because it's widely used, because people believe that unless it's a drunk driving accident you don't really die from it," says Phyllis Randall, a former mental health therapist who worked for over a decade treating offenders with substance abuse problems in an adult detention center.

Thousands of people out there, those who abuse alcohol and those who don't, are equally unaware of the fact that a longtime drinker can literally die when he or she gives up alcohol for good. Alcohol withdrawal is a very serious condition. *New York Times* bestselling crime author and Hollywood film writer Lowell Cauffiel made the dangerous decision to detox from alcohol on his own in order to feel the full result of withdrawal so as to never be tempted to drink again. At first, he felt like "his guts were being pulled out." Then he shook, had sweats and suffered vivid hallucinations. His experiment worked. Cauffiel hasn't had a drink since, but doctors said detoxing on his own could have killed him.

Coming off alcohol has resulted in the deaths of thousands. One example of this is the sad case of Nelsan Ellis, an American actor and playwright who achieved critical acclaim for his portrayal of Lafayette Reynolds in the popular HBO television series *True Blood*. The 39-year-old entertainer died in July of 2017. When reports of his passing first surfaced, his manager stated that Ellis died of "complications with heart failure". However, it wouldn't be long before the world realized the story behind the heart failure was much darker and more disturbing.

A few days after his initial statement, his manager let the world know the whole story behind Ellis' sudden death. The heart failure was caused by the actor's attempt to stop abusing alcohol on his own. The subsequent withdrawal is what led to his early demise. The actor's father reported that "after many stints in rehab, Nelsan attempted to withdraw from alcohol on his own."

People who try to quit drinking on their own run the risk of having a seizure, which often proves deadly. Not only is the alcoholic putting his or her life in jeopardy, but also the lives of others. One tragic example of this involved a man from the Tampa, Florida area. On the day after Christmas in 2017, the individual, who had suffered from years of alcohol abuse, decided to quit drinking cold turkey in order to improve his relationship with his significant other. That morning he got behind the wheel and, while driving, suffered a seizure that resulted from alcohol withdrawal. He slammed into another car, killing a 57-year-old woman.

The man, who decided to detox from alcohol on his own, which resulted in the death of an innocent woman, was charged with vehicular homicide. Prosecutors concluded that he should have known that a seizure was possible when he quit drinking, however he ignored this fact and decided to drive despite the risk. Now he runs the risk of spending time in prison, and the deceased woman's family has been robbed of their loved one.

As has been shown, trying to detox from alcohol without medical attention is extremely dangerous, especially if the person has been drinking for a long period of time. *WebMD* stated, "Alcohol withdraw syndrome is a potentially life-threatening condition that can occur in people who have been drinking heavily for weeks, months or years and then either stop or significantly reduce their alcohol consumption. Dying this way is not rare, in fact it happens more often than many people may realize. *WebMD* noted, "When heavy drinkers suddenly stop or significantly reduce their alcohol consumption, the neurotransmitters previously suppressed by alcohol are no longer suppressed. They rebound, resulting in a phenomenon known as brain hyperexcitability."

Symptoms of alcohol withdrawal can begin as early as two hours after the last drink. The most extreme and frightening alcohol withdrawal symptom is called delirium tremens, also knowns as "DTs," which I briefly mentioned earlier. It can be deadly. About 5% of people with alcohol withdrawal get delirium tremens. This is another reason why those in the addiction field recommend people detox from alcohol under medical supervision rather than attempting it on their own.

A famous 19th Century Russian composer by the name of Modest Mussorgsky is believed to have died as a result of delirium tremens. He was a skilled pianist, born into a wealthy family not far from what was then the nation's capital, St. Petersburg. Mussorgsky had much success in the world of music, which included operas. However, in his later years he was known to spend most of his days frequenting bars. By the time he reached his fifth decade, he had descended so far into his addiction that he landed in the hospital after suffering multiple seizures. He stopped drinking, and for a brief period of time it appeared his health was rebounding. Sadly however, that turned out to not be the case. The damage from alcoholism was irreversible and had taken an unforgiving toll. He died on March 28, 1881, just a few days after his 42nd birthday. The cause of death was delirium tremens.

So, what exactly is delirium tremens? Basically, it is an extreme reaction to alcohol withdrawal that is characterized by a severely confused state, disorientation, seizures and even hallucinations. The name delirium tremens was first used in the early 1800's; however, the symptoms were well described at least a century before. The symptoms of DTs can appear quickly; however, they usually don't develop for two to three days after a person's last drink.

For decades, characters suffering from delirium tremens have made their way into our books, movies and television shows. The famous 19th Century American author Mark Twain, who penned the well-known book *The Adventures of Huckleberry Finn*, described Huck's father as having suffering from this side effect of alcohol withdrawal. In chapter six, after guzzling whiskey,

Huck's father runs around with hallucinations of snakes and chases Huck around their cabin with a knife in an attempt to kill him, thinking Huck is the "Angel of Death."

More recently, storylines involving delirium tremens have been included in film and on the small screen. Entertainer Ray Milland won an Academy Award for Best Actor for portraying a character going through delirium tremens in the 1945 movie *The Lost World*. In the film, he hallucinates, believing he saw a bat fly in his hospital room and attack a rodent. The popular 1970's television show *M*A*S*H* also covered this serious topic. In one episode, a nurse was discovered to be drinking heavily when not at work. Two days later she became hysterical when served food, claiming that objects were crawling onto her from the plate. Another character recognized the symptoms of delirium tremens and ordered medication to aid the nurse's withdrawal.

These descriptions and portrayals of delirium tremens are frighteningly accurate. Hallucinations that result from it are terrifying. Before I knew what this alcohol withdrawal side effect was, I observed someone go through it. What I saw alarmed me. The male friend, 29 years old at the time, had been a heavy daily drinker for about five years at that point. On New Year's Eve he decided to stop drinking cold turkey. Over the course of the next several days he shook, he had seizures, he had a wild look in his eye, and he had frightening hallucinations. He ripped up a bathroom wall imaging rats were behind it.

I had never witnessed such a thing before, and I was convinced that he was lying to me when he said he was just coming off alcohol. I thought for sure hardcore street drugs were involved as well. I later learned that he was being truthful when he said it was just alcohol he was withdrawing from. That's how dangerous this toxic liquid is. If I had known exactly what he was going through then, I would have seen to it that he detoxed under medical supervision. However, I lacked the knowledge at the time to know he needed professional help. The mortality rate from delirium tremens without treatment is between 15% and 40%. He is lucky to be alive.

I've never seen, let alone touched, an illegal drug in my entire life. I knew, even as a young teenager, that getting hooked on a substance like heroin to "help" me cope with my problems would mean I just had one more problem. However, it never crossed my mind that if I drank to erase the mental pain, then that would also be just one more dilemma I would eventually have to tackle. It never crossed my mind because alcohol is legal, and heroin is not. It never crossed my mind because commercials advertise the "benefits" of drinking. It never crossed my mind because television sitcoms and movies glamourize characters who consume alcohol. Therefore, it never crossed my mind that alcohol was a drug, just like heroin, until it was almost too late.

Yes, alcohol is a drug, and it's the most dangerous drug in the world.

CHAPTER 4:

Alcohol And Our Health

When I first realized I needed to control my drinking, my goal was just that, to control it. I didn't intend to stop entirely. I thought, "Yes I need to stop self-medicating, but come on, when I travel to exotic countries, I want to try the local beers and wines." Of course, we have already touched on the fact that alcohol advertisements have seeped into our subconscious, making us believe we NEED to drink to enjoy our vacations when that simply isn't true. This helped me stop drinking altogether, but so did the realization of what alcohol actually is.

So, what exactly is alcohol? If you had asked me that question just a few years ago, I would have naively answered, "Well beer is wheat, vodka is from potatoes and wine comes from grapes!" I would have responded this way because that is what I had been led to believe all of my life, that alcohol is derived from the healthy foods we eat every day. So, if alcohol comes from what we eat, it can't be that bad for our bodies, right? Boy, was I ever wrong!

In chapter seven of *This Naked Mind*, Annie Grace wrote, "I had assumed it was common knowledge that alcohol is harmful to your health. I was wrong. More than seven thousand people volunteered to be beta readers – reading early drafts of the book and providing feedback during the editing process. As their comments poured in, I realized that it is not common knowledge that alcohol is harmful. In fact, we have been so indoctrinated that we believe the opposite is true. Common knowledge actually claims that moderate drinking defined as one to three drinks per day, benefits our health."

Have you heard that wine is good for your heart? Have you touted an article that you read which claimed having a few drinks per week benefits your health? I know I have. I read one article about alcohol being "good for you" and ran with it, perhaps as an excuse to keep drinking. Meanwhile I ignored the countless other articles that stated the actual facts, that alcohol is a toxic liquid that causes cancer, heart failure and liver damage. Why then, do the few articles on the supposed health benefits of drinking grab our attention and stay in our memories while the hundreds of scientifically backed ones that prove alcohol leads to severe bodily problems get pushed aside? Grace sums it up in her book.

It's the job of a journalist to write attention-grabbing articles, ones that people will read, share with others and discuss. As Grace states, "This enables them to claim a higher readership, sell more advertisements, and build their business." There are countless studies that prove the dangers that come along with drinking alcohol, but there are fewer articles about these studies because journalists know those articles won't sell well in our culture. Grace backed this fact up when she did a

Google search on the subject. She searched "alcohol harms" and "alcohol dangers" and the instant results included studies from the National Institute of Alcohol Abuse and Alcoholism. It also included medical sites like *WebMD*. However, when she searched both of those terms, it did not lead to a single popular publication. When she searched "alcohol healthy," no reliable articles appeared, however she was bombarded by popular yet unscientific articles with headlines that boosted the "benefits" of drinking.

This is one reason we have duped ourselves into believing drinking can be good for us, despite all the scientific evidence that has been proven against this claim. And we repeat what the journalists print. Think about it, how many times have you been on social media and have seen a friend post a positive article about alcohol verses a negative one? I'm willing to bet the "good" articles far outweigh the bad. What if I shared an article on Facebook that claimed red wine was good for the heart? I'm willing to bet it would get a lot of "likes." What if I had instead shared a scientific article from a respectable medical journal about the dangers of drinking? My guess is few would "like" that post.

So, are there any benefits to alcohol? Well, it is an antiseptic, which is applied to living tissue/skin to reduce the possibility of infection. In other words, it can be used to dull physical pain. But then again, so can ibuprofen. In fact, doctors claim ibuprofen is better than alcohol in this regard. What about the supposed health benefits of drinking wine? According to *This Naked Mind*, "A new study that analyzed the drinking habits and cardiovascular health of over 260,000 people shows that drinking alcohol, even in moderate amounts, provides no heart-health benefit."

So, what exactly is alcohol made from? Remember what I wrote earlier, how I had believed well into my thirties that beer is wheat, vodka is potatoes and wine is derived from grapes? I thought it was pretty straight forward and simple. I had no idea that alcohol is ethanol, a chemical compound. Ethanol is a flammable, colorless liquid that is poisonous. This is why I now refer to alcohol as a "toxic liquid," because that is exactly what it is. The alcohol you drink at parties, happy hours and at dinner is the exact same liquid that you pump into your vehicle to make it run. Yes, that is what you are drinking. I initially wanted to cut back on my drinking, to stop using it to self-medicate. However, when I realized that I was guzzling the same substance that I use to fuel my car, my desire to drink completely evaporated.

According to page 60 of *This Naked Mind*, "The World Health Organization (WHO) states that 'alcohol is a casual factor in sixty types of diseases and injuries.' The report goes on to say that alcohol has surpassed AIDS and is now the world's leading risk factor for death among males 15-59." *This Naked Mind* goes on to state that researchers evaluated numerous drugs to learn their overall harm on the user and those they come into contact with. Alcohol scored as the most harmful drug, proving even worse than heroin and crack cocaine.

This is serious. Alcohol is much more dangerous than the average person realizes. The damage alcohol does to the human body is horrifying. Let's look at the facts that surround the toll drinking takes on the brain, the heart and the liver, as well as the human nervous system.

WebMD reports, "Thirty seconds after your first sip, alcohol races into your brain. It slows down the chemicals and pathways that your brain cells use to send messages. That alters your mood, slows your reflexes, and throws off your balance. You also can't think straight, which you may not recall later, because you'll struggle to store things in long-term memory." Drinking can actually shrink the brain, which in turn makes it hard to learn and remember. Those who start drinking at an early age, particularly the teen years, and those who drink heavily for a long period of their lives, are the most at risk for this kind of destruction. Maria Pagano, PhD., addiction researcher and professor of psychiatry at Case Western Reserve University School of Medicine, states that drinking alcohol alters the level of neurotransmitters in the brain. "For starters, alcohol slows down the neurotransmitters GABA, and that's what drives the sluggish movements, slurred speech and slower reaction time in someone who's intoxicated," she says. Also, binge drinking can result in damage in the limbic system that occurs after a relatively short period of time. This means you don't necessarily have to have been drinking for a long period in your life to do this kind of destruction. It's daunting to think about, but this brain damage increases the risk of dementia, as well as abnormalities in mood and cognitive abilities.

The wine that we have been led to believe is so good for the heart can do its fair share of damage as well. According to the *Mayo Clinic*, "it's possible that red wine isn't any better than beer, white wine or liquor for heart health. There's still no clear evidence that red wine is better than other forms of alcohol when it comes to possible heart-healthy benefits." The truth is, consuming alcohol can lead to a heart attack because of extensive damage to the cardiovascular system. In fact numerous studies have found that, after taking into account other risk factors such as being overweight or smoking, drinking increases the risk of a heart attack by 40 percent. Wine, including red wine, is not some miracle beverage that can cure the heart.

Let's move on to the liver. We've all heard that over time, too much alcohol can damage this important organ. The liver is vital to the human body because when harmful toxins and substances enter your blood stream, your liver acts fast to detoxify and destroy them. It filters the blood, which removes dead cells and harmful bacteria. Toxins are then quickly transported to your intestine or your kidneys for disposal. This is why it is so important to maintain a healthy liver, which alcohol is known to destroy. In fact, you might be surprised to learn that two million Americans suffer alcohol-related liver disease.

Alcohol liver disease used to be considered "an old man disease," according to Jessica Mellinger, M.D. Now it is affecting all age groups, young and old, and women are especially at risk. Females absorb and metabolize alcohol differently from males, which makes that gender more susceptible to liver damage. More and more mothers are drinking, and they laugh about needing wine, which has been nicknamed "mommy juice." Mellinger states, "There is this 'mommy juice' culture, this 'mommy juice' humor involving wine that's normalizing drinking in a bad way. There is nothing funny about alcoholic liver disease.

When I lived and worked in DC in my late 20's, I met a young woman my age who I eventually formed a friendship with. When the topic of our families came up, she would sometimes mention that her father abused alcohol. I didn't think much of it. Apparently, she didn't either. We were young professionals then, going to happy hours after work and spending our Friday nights drinking the time away at local clubs. About a year after we met, her father's liver finally started to fail. Years of drinking had caught up to him, and he lost his life to it. My friend was, of course, devastated by her loss. However, I look back at that time now and realize her father's death did not make her question her drinking. She continued to consume alcohol like she had before, never mentioning that maybe she should stop or else her life could be in jeopardy, too.

When researching people who have passed due to the damage alcohol took on their livers, I came across an article about a young British woman named Amy. Her sister died of complications associated with liver disease just before her 28th birthday. "It really shocked me how quickly she deteriorated," Amy said. Her sister, depressed after a breakup, started to drink heavily in her early 20's. After that, it spiraled out of control. "Two years before she passed away, doctors told us that she was terminally ill," said Amy. "They said nothing could be done to save her and told us that, going forward, it was just about managing her treatments."

Amy's sister never lived to see the age of 30. She died young and in pain, all because she had abused alcohol. Sadly, she is one of countless people who lose their lives this way every year. What's even more tragic is the fact that dying this way is completely avoidable. It doesn't have to happen.

It is not surprising that drinking also affects our immune systems in a profoundly negative way. People who drink on a regular basis may notice that they are more prone to catching a cold, the flu or other diseases than their peers who don't regularly consume alcohol. This is because alcohol makes the body more susceptible to illness and infections. Also, abusing alcohol can result in other conditions, such as leaky gut syndrome, which allows bacteria from the bowel to seep or "leak" through the walls of the intestines. Harmful bacteria can cause infections.

Many may not realize that drinking alcohol can lead to many different types of cancers. According to Laura A. Stokowski, RN, "Responsible drinking has become a 21st Century mantra for how most people view alcohol consumption. But when it comes to cancer, no amount of alcohol is safe." Yes, you read that right. Even a small amount of alcohol can lead to this deadly disease we hear and read so much about. Page 67 of *This Naked Mind* states, "A seven-year-study of 1.2 million middle-aged women highlights the direct and terrifying link between drinking and cancer. According to this study, alcohol increased the chance of developing cancers of the breast, mouth, throat, rectum, liver and esophagus." What is perhaps most startling is that cancer risk increases no matter how much we drink and no matter the choice of alcohol. Even small amounts can cause cancer to develop.

So how exactly does drinking lead to this devastating disease? The Centers for Disease Control and Prevention sums it up perfectly. "When you drink alcohol, your body breaks it down into a chemical called acetaldehyde. Acetaldehyde damages your DNA and prevents your body from repairing the damage. DNA is the cell's "instruction manual" that controls a cell's normal growth and function. When DNA is damaged, a cell can begin growing out of control and create a cancer tumor."

Anyone who drinks is at risk of coming down with some form of cancer. It doesn't matter if you are male or female. Rich or poor. A celebrity or not. Cancer doesn't discriminate. Millions are familiar with the name Mickey Mantle, the famous New York Yankees center fielder. He was a huge success; he was the highest-paid active player of his time. Tragically, fame and success did not protect him from the horrors of alcoholism.

In 1994, Mantel checked into a treatment center to help him overcome his addiction after being told by a doctor that his liver was badly damaged after nearly four decades of drinking. The doctor also told Mantle that the damage inflicted by alcohol to his system was so severe that "your next drink could be your last." As he neared the end of his life, the famous baseball player who was admired by thousands stated that he regretted all the years he drank. Alcohol, he admitted, had often caused him to act cruelly towards his family, friends and his fans. Doctors eventually discovered he had an inoperable type of liver cancer. The baseball legend succumbed to this disease, caused by years of alcohol abuse. It was a dismal ending to a once admired and respected life.

With every drink we take, we are putting ethanol into our bodies and putting our health, which we often take for granted, at risk. There are practically no health benefits to drinking, yet there are more than enough ways that downing that can of beer or sipping that glass of wine can lead to devasting, life-long health issues. Next time you consider taking a drink, think to yourself, is it really worth jeopardizing my health?

CHAPTER 5:

What Alcohol Takes Away

Alcohol steals from us. It steals our health, our memories, our time and our money. It steals our homes and our jobs. Perhaps worse of all, it steals our families, our friends and our futures. This toxic liquid is not a positive companion. It is a sneaky foe, pretending that we need it to enjoy life, to be happy, to relax, to squash our anxieties and our fears. Instead alcohol is a wolf in sheep's clothing. It causes diseases, heartache and misery. So many people have lost so much due to their alcohol abuse. I was fortunate enough to escape the total downfall, but I came very, very close to losing everything.

Countless people every day across the country and the world witness sad cases of those who have lost their jobs, every loving family member and every possession they own due to drinking. They sit on street corners, begging for money so they can buy a six pack of beer or another bottle of vodka. Getting their next "fix," their next drink, is the addicts only concern.

I see it all the time when walking the streets of the city I currently reside in. In fact, just two days ago, I witnessed a police officer encounter with a homeless man that broke my heart and nearly made my eyes tear. I was walking to a nearby grocery store when I caught a portion of the conversation between the two. The homeless man wore tattered clothes. His face was dirty, and his hair was caked with mud. It was clear the man had not had a decent shower in a very, very long time. There was a can of beer under the bench where he was sitting. The police officer was trying to talk the man out of his sad, pathetic situation. "Wouldn't you rather get help than live out here?" the officer asked. The homeless man didn't respond. By the time I had finished my shopping and passed back by 30 minutes later, the officer was gone, and the homeless man was still sitting in the same spot, the beer can within reach. And it was in that moment I realized that was almost me.

Just one month earlier, I had a direct encounter with a woman who had lost it all due to addiction. It was Valentine's Day, and that evening I decided to enjoy the warm, Florida night outside. I was a bit upset that I wasn't spending the time with the person I loved, who was away that night. So, I decided to put my headphones on and listen to some soothing music while taking an evening stroll. My walk led me to a local playground. I sat down on a swing and gazed up at the starry sky.

When my gaze turned back down towards earth, I looked to my side and noticed a woman preparing a sleeping bag under a bench. She saw me and asked me my name. After I replied, she informed me her name was Cindy. She then said that she had been living in a halfway house, but had failed a drug test, so she was kicked out of the facility. This woman's addiction had caused her to lose everything, even a spot in a crummy halfway house!

After we chatted, I ran back to my residence, grabbed a bag of fresh bagels and went back to the park to deliver them to her. I knew not to give her money, as she would likely just spend it at the nearby liquor store. However, I wanted to provide her with some food in an attempt to make her realize that a total stranger cared about her, perhaps prompting her to realize that she had value and could give up the addiction and win her life back.

Sadly, these are just two examples of people who lost it all due to drinking. There are thousands of cases every year in which successful, promising people fall so far into their alcohol addiction that nothing else matters except getting their next drink, even if it means that they must live on the streets.

Let's look at the sad story of a man from Great Britain by the name of Kevin. He grew up with an alcoholic father and swore that, while he enjoyed drinking, he would never follow in his father's footsteps. Kevin spent a great deal of time at his local pub. His wife soon became angry about this fact, to which Kevin's response was to just come join him in a night of drinking, she didn't have to stay home alone. Usually this suggestion would result in an argument, in which Kevin would leave and then return home later that night intoxicated. His wife eventually filed for divorce, but Kevin still refused to acknowledge that he was going down the same destructive path as his father.

After a couple years, and a few run-ins with the law, Kevin's drinking only got worse. He blamed it on the divorce and the fact he was trying to block out the pain. Like a lot of people, Kevin was using alcohol to self-medicate. Soon, his friends started avoiding him. Eventually, he lost everything good in his life and decided he needed to get help or else he would die. After regaining his life after years of alcohol abuse, Kevin remarked on the cold, hard facts of drinking in order to self-medicate. "They say alcohol is a great remover; how true! I lost everything and was now homeless. Every penny I could lay my hands on went to cheap white cider."

It isn't just your average, every day person who can lose everything to drinking. The horrific results of alcohol abuse do not discriminate. Anyone can fall victim. In fact, countless celebrities have seen their fame and fortune evaporate due to alcohol abuse.

Today, most people do not recognize the name Mary Pickford, however she played a crucial role in creating the movie industry as we know it today, and she did so at a time when women weren't even allowed to vote. As a young adult, she was one of the original founders of the Academy of Motion Picture Arts and Sciences and one of the most popular actresses of the 1910's and 1920's. The curly-haired brunette was awarded the second ever Academy Award for Best Actress in 1929, and by the close of the 20th Century, the American Film Institute ranked her as the 24th greatest female star of classic Hollywood cinema.

Despite her success in pioneering the movie industry, Pickford's latter years would be filled with heartache. The end of the silent film era left Pickford deeply depressed. As her star faded into obscurity and she eventually retired, the once vibrant entertainer turned to drinking, just like her father had done before her. Both of her siblings, who had also been successful in the acting world, passed away from alcohol-related causes. Pickford died a recluse at the age of 87.

In 2014, one hundred years after she helped create Hollywood as we now know it, an online article came out chronicling Pickford's life, success and death. At the bottom of the page, a 21st Century fan left a comment reflecting on the actress' finals days. He wrote, "A sad life behind the scenes. Her father was an alcoholic, her first husband was and after her divorce from (Douglas) Fairbanks, the two children she adopted later became alcoholics, and in the end she did. It wasn't all roses and success." Drinking ruined this entire once successful, early Hollywood family.

Alcohol abuse has not only destroyed or threatened to destroy those who found fame in the entertainment industry. Well-known politicians have also been negatively affected by drinking, as well as their families.

The Betty Ford Center is universally known to millions. Founded by former First Lady of the United States, Betty Ford, it helps countless people overcome their addiction to alcohol every year. After her husband, President Gerald Ford, lost his re-election campaign for Commander in Chief in 1976, her family staged an intervention and forced her to confront her alcoholism. "I liked alcohol," she wrote years later in her memoir. "It made me feel warm." She went into treatment for substance abuse. By the 1980's she had recovered and opened the treatment center that bears her name.

Barbara Bush, one of Ford's successors as First Lady, stated that Ford, "transformed her pain into something great for the common good. Because she suffered, there will be more healing. Because of her grief, there will be more joy." Unlike movie legend

Mary Pickford, Ford's alcohol story ended on a much better note. She beat an addiction that ruins millions. She succeeded. She survived.

Betty Ford is certainly not the only bright, uplifting story to come out of the dark clutches of alcohol addiction. Actress Drew Barrymore, who descends from Hollywood royalty, is another one. She is a well-known movie star to Generation X and Millennial audiences, and was honored by the Young Artist Foundation with its Former Child Star "Lifetime Achievement" Award. Five years later, she received a motion picture star on the Hollywood Walk of Fame in 2004. Today she is a happy mother of two and continues to have success in the entertainment industry. However, life wasn't always like this for the actress.

Barrymore comes from a long line of successful Hollywood entertainers, who in turn were all riddled with the curse of alcohol addiction. Dating back to the early days of the movie industry, the Barrymores made a name for themselves. Ironically, her grandfather, John Barrymore, was a friend of Mary Pickford during the Silent Era. Like Pickford, he had a serious issue with drinking. As his alcohol dependency grew, studios were less willing to employ him despite his popularity with movie viewers. Today, decades after his passing, he is perhaps more remembered for his drinking than his acting.

For a while, it seemed like his granddaughter, Drew, would go down the same destructive path. She exploded on the entertainment scene at the tender age of seven when she was cast as a main character in the blockbuster hit, E.T. That same year she became the youngest person to host the popular comedy show *Saturday Night Live*, in which the first grader joked about her family's history of alcohol abuse. Sadly, it was during this time that the child was being exposed to alcohol in real life. By her teen years she was making headlines as a "troubled child" with her underage drinking and partying ways.

However, once she reached her 20's, the actress decided to turn her life around and avoided the fate of famous family members who had gone before her. Barrymore starred in several box office hits, and by the dawn of 21st Century, she had gained an excellent reputation among Hollywood directors to work with. She is proof that just because someone comes from a long line of alcohol abusers doesn't mean that person is doomed to follow in their footsteps. Recovery is possible for everyone out there.

How does one escape the trap of addiction when he or she has a family history of heavy drinking? If a person can date alcohol abuse going back generations, isn't that individual doomed to drinking from the start? While this might be a common belief among many, the truth is no one has to repeat family history. I have mentioned author Annie Grace and her incredibly insightful piece of work *This Naked Mind* several times throughout this book. She is one example of a person who broke free from the chains of alcohol abuse and, interestingly enough, so did her father.

Grace mentions in her book that her father, who had been a drinker for most of her life, woke up one day and decided that alcohol needed to be cut from his life entirely. According to Grace, "I never knew my dad to drink, so I assumed he never had. In reality, he was known for his heavy drinking and drank as much or more than any other fraternity boy in the '60s." So, what made him stop cold turkey? Grace states that one day he had a simple epiphany. He remarked, "I realized it wasn't doing me any favors, so I decided to stop. I never looked back." He continues to live an alcohol-free existence to this day.

Despite having a father who used to be alcohol dependent, Grace, too, has freed herself from a life that consisted of daily drinking. Her alcohol abuse started early as a young professional when she felt like she had to drink in order to fit in and prove herself to her drinking colleagues. She once told me that, at her worst, she was drinking two bottles of wine a night. However, when she finally decided to take a step back and re-evaluate her relationship with alcohol, she realized her drinking was out of control. After much research and producing her amazing book that has helped countless people, myself included, she quit drinking altogether and has become an inspiration to those who wish to remove this toxic liquid from their lives.

Alcohol is not your friend. Despite what you have been led to believe, it does not help to relax you in stressful situations. It does not give you "liquid courage." It does not make an already good time even better. Most importantly, it does not solve your problems. Instead alcohol leads to heartache, misery and death. It leads to jails and institutions. It causes admired, promising, successful people to lose everything good in their lives, including their jobs, families and close friends. It ruins people's finances and causes homelessness. Alcohol takes, and it does not give anything good in return. It poisons our bodies and harms our minds. It is a sneaky enemy that ruins everything positive in our lives.

I once came across a saying that sums up alcohol perfectly. It's something to remember if the temptation to drink ever arises, especially if a person uses alcohol to self-medicate. The saying goes:

> *At first, alcohol will take away your pain.*
> *Then it will take your joy, your freedom and your family.*
> *It will take away your home, your job and your self-respect.*
> *Eventually it will take away everything and you will be*
> *left will nothing but the pain you were trying to escape.*

CHAPTER 6

A Worldwide Epidemic: Part 1

Alcohol Use Disorder is a worldwide epidemic. In fact, alcohol is taking more lives every year than opioids, despite the latter receiving far more media attention. According to the World Health Organization (WHO), there are over 3 million deaths globally every year resulting from the harmful use of alcohol. A 2018 online article from *Medical News Today* describes Alcohol Use Disorder as a "chronic relapsing brain disease" where a person drinks compulsively, often to the point of it interfering with their daily life. It is a condition in which a person has a desire or physical need to consume alcohol, even though it has a negative impact on their life.

In all six of the continents people populate, drinking is a leading health concern. Of all the countries in the world, the top five nations where drinking is at its worse are found in Eastern Europe, including Russia. The other four are Belarus, Moldova,

Lithuania and Romania. Rounding out the top ten are Ukraine, Andorra, Hungary, Czech Republic and Slovakia.

The countries where Alcohol Use Disorder are all but nonexistent are mostly nations found in the Middle East, where drinking is strictly forbidden by devote Muslims. The top ten nations where alcohol is not a severe issue are Egypt, Niger, Yemen, Comoros, Saudi Arabia, Bangladesh, Kuwait, Libya, Mauritania and Pakistan. In many of these nations, simply consuming alcohol can result in severe punishments by the governments.

In the next two chapters, I examine each continent's dependency on alcohol, why drinking has become such an epidemic and if the tide might (hopefully) soon change. This chapter is dedicated to the Western Hemisphere; North and South America. Some facts regarding alcohol use in the countries that make up these continents may surprise many.

Canada is one of the northernmost countries in the world, and the second largest. It consists of ten provinces and three territories, and stretches from the Atlantic to Pacific Oceans and northward to the Arctic. Despite its vast size, it is a nation of only 37,314,442. In 2016, it was reported that 19% of Canadians aged 12 and older were considered heavy drinkers. This is nearly 6 million of the population.

According to the website *Alcohol Rehab*, alcohol is the most abused drug in Canada. Overall, it is believed that citizens are likely drinking less now than they did in previous decades, but alcohol abuse continues to be a significant issue. Binge drinking is on the rise, and underage drinking continues to be a problem.

Approximately 2,000 people die each year as a result of alcoholic liver disease in Canada, with the heaviest drinking taking place in Quebec and Newfoundland.

The good news is, that despite Alcohol Use Disorder still affecting so many Canadian citizens, drinking does seem to be on the decline across that nation. One reason may be that a DUI conviction in Canada runs the risk of a felony, causing many to reconsider their drinking habits. Another likely possibility for the reduction of alcohol consumption is education; people are more aware of the health risk that comes with excessive drinking compared to previous decades.

"While we still have work to do, particularly with young people, things are evolving in a positive direction and our efforts are bearing fruit," said Hubert Sacy, Director General of Éduc'alcool, a nonprofit organization that seeks to help people make positive decisions involving drinking responsibly. Its slogan is "Moderation is always in good taste."

Canada's neighbor to the south, the United States, may also be seeing a decrease in alcohol consumption, though it remains a problematic issue there as well. According to the National Institute on Alcohol Abuse and Alcoholism, an estimated 16 million Americans suffer from Alcohol Use Disorder. Approximately 15 million adults ages 18 and older suffer from this issue, and over 600,000 people under 17 do as well. These are staggering numbers in a nation of 327 million people, the world's third most populous country.

However, as stated before, there are signs that Americans are beginning to scale back their drinking habits. Perhaps surprisingly, Millennials (those born between 1980 and 1995) is the age group drinking less. Why is this? A 2017 *Forbes* article, penned by Jules Schroeder, provided her opinion of this hopeful trend. "For Millennials today, it's become somewhat of a faux pas to drink. While our parents' generation considered booze cool, we think it the opposite. Instead, connection, authenticity, and mindfulness are what's catching on, and as a result, producing many benefits," she stated.

Unlike previous generations, others in this age range are now considering the numerous risk that comes along with excessive drinking. "I drank pretty regularly in my 20s, especially in social situations," Leanne Vanderbyl, of San Francisco, said. "It wasn't until I hit my 30s that I realized that alcohol was no longer my friend." She isn't alone in her thoughts. Amanda Mull, a writer for *The Atlantic*, interviewed more than 100 Americans in their 20's and 30's, the subject being alcohol consumption. All "have begun to make similar changes in their drinking habits or who are contemplating ways to drink less."

According to Mull, Generation Z (those born after 1995) could see an even greater decrease in drinkers. Data has shown much lower rates for alcohol consumption among those in their teens and early 20's. This is in stark contrast to previous generations.

It seems that restaurants across the country are picking up on this positive trend. *The San Francisco Chronicle* produced an article in 2019 that covered the fact that more and more Bay Area bars are serving alcohol-free "mocktails" due to popular demand. "Dry January," a term used to describe ditching alcohol in the first month of the new year, is an annual tradition for countless people, and it continues to grow in popularity with each passing year. In honor of this, bars throughout the city of Chicago serve up drinks that contain zero percent alcohol. "We wanted to have dynamic drink options for people who don't want to drink," reported Danny Shapiro in a 2018 *Chicago Tribune* article. He is a partner and beverage director of Scofflaw Group's zero-alcohol offerings at The Moonlighter, located in the Windy City.

We can remain hopeful that this non-drinking trend will continue in the United States. If it does, Millennials, members of Generation Z and future generations will escape the financial and physical pain drinking has brought to previous generations. No doubt alcohol-related cancers will go down across the country, and the population will continue to grow healthier. It is a positive outlook for what is (with any luck) to come.

Going further south to Mexico and Central America, alcohol consumption is a way of life for millions. In Mexico alone, at least 70% of the population drinks, and 20% does so in excess. Unlike the United States, where alcohol use among the young seems to be decreasing in numbers, the same can not be said about those south of the border. In Mexico, alcohol consumption in excess has steadily risen among minors between 12 and 17 years old. According to a 2014 survey, more than 70 percent of high school students have already had their first drink, and more than 15 percent drink excessively.

Underage alcohol use in Mexico has resulted in rising crime rates, and a recent study found that males were significantly more likely than females to be heavy drinkers, although female drinking rates have increased over time. Among those college age, males were more likely than females to report problems with friends, or encountering a physical fight because they drank. On a somewhat good note, the majority of students (70 percent) fell into the "infrequent" and "occasional" category when it comes to drinking, meaning a vast majority do not abuse the substance. However, over 20 percent were "regular drinkers," over 6 percent were "heavy drinkers, and nearly 2 percent drink is excess.

In Central America, a region that is riddled with poverty and high crime, citizens depend on alcohol in an attempt to "escape" their dire living conditions. Many, lacking the knowledge that alcohol is a depressant, rely on it in hopes of relaxing or feeling better, unaware they are making their situations worse. According to the website *Central America Data*, "Panama is the country where the highest proportion of beer consumption was reported with respect to total alcohol consumed, with 77%, followed by Costa Rica and Guatemala, with 64% and 56%, respectively."

The same website stated that alcohol consumption was on the rise in Costa Rico. This may come as a surprise to many, as it is often viewed as the most "stable" of all the Central American countries. Between 2009 and 2013 wine sales grew by 77%, followed by vodka, which increased by 43%, whiskey 38% and rum 31%. During the 2010's, distribution in bars, restaurants, and grocery and liquor stores increased by 32%.

Perhaps in an attempt to curb drinking in the region among locals and vacationers, tourism agencies and websites are encouraging people to opt for non-alcoholic drinks. One website highlights the fact that Central America is known for its coffees, and highlights the fact that you can do a tour of the production facilities. The same website also mentions other non-alcoholic beverages that are gaining traction in several of those countries, including Limonade con soda, seaweed shakes and Refresco, made from fruits including coconut, pineapple and mango.

Panama is also making attempts to reduce alcohol consumption among its population. By enacting new laws, the country hopes that drinking will decrease. On March 1, 2018 the government started to enforce nine "Spring Break" laws to control excessive public drinking at popular beaches. The laws include making beaches alcohol-free zones, prohibiting open house parties and no alcohol is permitted in parking lots. In March, when spring break typically occurs, alcohol sales end at 2 am.

The island nations that make up the Caribbean also have a problem with excessive drinking among their populations, where unlike the United States, the drinking age is 18. However, unlike other countries in North America, these nations don't seem to be attempting to better the issue of Alcohol Use Disorder among their citizens. It is a disturbing and frightening fact that it is not illegal to drive while under the influence in most of the islands. It is commonplace to see people driving with a can of beer in their hands or drinking while talking to a policeman on a beach or along the side of a road.

It has been reported that there are more rum shops than churches in some countries in the Caribbean. In 2012, the small country of Grenada ranked 16th overall in the global alcohol consumption. The Bahamas, a popular cruise destination for many Americans and others across the world, came in at number 8. There does not appear to be much attempt to decrease alcohol consumption in this part of the world. Sadly, it doesn't seem to be a concern for most of its citizens. Drinking is so prevalent in the islands among the locals and vacationers, that life without it seems unfathomable.

As we can see from researching the countries that make up North America, alcohol consumption is on the rise in some areas, whereas it is decreasing in others. In the nations where drinking has grown, citizens will hopefully become more educated in the coming years in regard to the dangers that come along with relying on this toxic liquid.

The countries that make up South America include (in alphabetical order) are Argentina, Bolivia, Brazil, Chile, Colombia, Ecuador, Guyana, Paraguay, Peru, Suriname, Uruguay, and Venezuela. Each has dealt with the negative impact that comes with drinking, and each are trying to combat this epidemic to avoid rising crime rates and increasing health problems.

Known for its many wines, it is perhaps not surprising that Argentina takes the award for the most alcohol consumption in this continent. Chile comes in second place, and Peru and Brazil are tied in the third position with each country having a consumption of 8.9 liters for those age 15 and older. In regard to Argentina, it is interesting to note that the World Health Organization has reported that the nation's alcohol consumption has been decreasing since the 1960's. This is, obviously, good news, however the fact remains that drinking has grown among females and adolescents. In an attempt to discourage underage drinking, the country has increased taxes on alcoholic beverages, hoping to make it more inaccessible for younger people.

Brazil, the largest country in South America in both size and population, is not known as one of the highest consumers of alcohol in the world. However, it has had its share of issues among its citizens who do drink. A 2013 research study found that alcohol consumption has increased over 30% with women and young people, and that 56% of all alcoholic drinks sold in the country are consumed by only 20% of the citizens who drink. The country is also dealing with a high rate of car accidents as a result of drunk driving, in which alcohol is linked to 21% of crashes. To combat this, a 2013 change in the law was made so that ANY amount of alcohol in the bloodstream of a driver who crashes his or her car is punishable.

In Chile, researchers are trying to tackle the problem of excessive drinking in a unique fashion. They are working diligently to come up with a vaccine against Alcohol Use Disorder. If successful, the patient will get a shot a month and not crave alcohol anymore. According to the website *Alcoholism Research*, "the vaccine would work like a cigarette patch, but would specifically target liver cells, he told the news service. The idea is to reduce the habit by 90 to 95 percent."

In both North and South America, Alcohol Use Disorder is a problem for many. Some nations may never attempt to tackle this issue, however as we have learned, other ones seem to be moving more and more to reducing the amount its citizens are taking in. The good news for places like the United States is that the move towards a more alcohol-free society is not the result of new laws and regulations, but due to people's personal choice, making the trend more likely to stick.

CHAPTER 7

A Worldwide Epidemic: Part 2

In the previous chapter, we looked at how alcohol has had a negative impact in the Western Hemisphere and how in nations such as the United States drinking is becoming less and less of a popular pastime. Now we move on to the Eastern Hemisphere and take a look at the role alcohol has in Africa, Asia, Australia and, of course, Europe. There are many similarities between the two hemispheres, and many differences as well.

Unlike the Western Hemisphere, where no country outright bans the use of alcohol, the same cannot be said about the Eastern Hemisphere. As I mentioned in the previous chapter, the countries where Alcohol Use Disorder are all but nonexistent are mostly nations found in the Middle East, where drinking is strictly forbidden by devote Muslims. Just consuming alcohol often results in severe punishments by many of these governments.

Some claim that the Quran discourages the use of alcohol, whereas others believe it does not. Whichever is true, the fact is several Middle Eastern nations have an across the board ban or make it so that only those who follow Islam can not drink. Perhaps the most well-known nation in this region with an outright ban for everyone, including tourist, is Saudi Arabia, home to the holy cities of Mecca and Medina. Drinking can be punishable by long prison sentences, public flogging or even execution.

In 2014, Karl Andree, a British national living in Saudi Arabia made international headlines when he was sentenced to jail time and 350 lashes for having home-brewed bottles of wine in his car. Andree, who was over 70 years old, spent over a year in jail before international outrage over his harsh sentences pressured the Saudi government to release him and he was allowed to fly back home to his native country. *The Guardian* reported in 2015 that he said his supporters had "saved my life" and added: "I am overwhelmed by the support and am grateful to prime minister David Cameron and the government for stepping in."

Others have not been as fortunate. The same year that Andree was released from the Saudi prison where he was held and allowed to return to the United Kingdom, a grandfather from Australia named Peter Mutty received prison time and given 28 strokes by a cane before being released on March 19 of that year. Of his time in the Saudi prison, Mutty said, "It was terrible, it was everything you imagine it would be. I was held with rapists, murderers and killers."

As mentioned before, other Middle Eastern nations do not have an outright ban of alcohol use like Saudi Arabia, but only prohibit their Muslim citizens from consuming the toxic liquid. In the United Arab Emirates, alcohol is allowed to be sold in restaurants, hotels and other places when the seller obtains a valid license. Non-Muslims who reside there are allowed to drink, but only in their private residences, hotels or bars they visit.

Perhaps surprising to some, many Middle Eastern nations have no ban on alcohol at all, despite their large Muslim populations. In Egypt, long known as a popular tourist destination with people all over the world due to its ancient pyramids and the famous Nile River, does not ban alcohol. Perhaps because tourism is, in many ways, Egypt's bread and butter, the government knew that banning this addictive substance would hurt the industry. Most natives who follow Islam chose not to drink in accordance to their beliefs, but if they do, they won't face jail time or other harsh punishments like in Saudi Arabia. However, drinking is expensive in Egypt, which is perhaps one reason why most people have not had much of a negative impact from it. They simply can't afford alcohol.

Outside the Middle East, a small number of African countries also have a complete ban on drinking. Since 1983, alcohol consumption has been illegal in Sudan when the Sudan Socialist Union passed the Liquor Prohibition Bill, making it illegal to manufacture, sell and drink the toxic liquid. In Somalia, located just across the famous Red Sea from Saudi Arabia, no one in the country can come in contact with alcohol. Though drinking was once allowed there, the Islamic government eventually put an end to that. In 2019, two Canadian women were jailed for several months for consuming alcohol, claiming they endured torture while being held. They were eventually freed.

In other parts of Africa, where Islam isn't the dominate religion, most people do not drink, yet Alcohol Use Disorder is still reportedly on the rise. However, this is being ignored by most policy-makers and the populations overall. In 2014, The *British Broadcasting Corporation (BBC)* reported a disturbing story in which 60 people died in Kenya after drinking homemade alcohol believed to have been laced with industrial chemicals, whereas dozens more were blinded. Homemade brewing is common in Kenya since most of its citizens cannot afford standardized alcohol. This is not the first time such a tragedy occurred there. Almost a decade earlier, more than 45 people died after drinking illegal alcohol laced with methanol.

The African country with the highest number of drinkers is by far Nigeria, where religious leaders are attempting to make it more difficult and expensive to produce and sell alcoholic beverages. One of the most popular drinks there is Ogogoro, which has a frighteningly high ethanol content of 30 to 60 percent! While there are 8 known breweries in Nigeria, most alcoholic drinks are home-made, perhaps for economic reasons like in Kenya. Not surprisingly, medical experts say alcohol dependency has led to a rise in diseases and has done much to contribute to Nigeria's grim road safety statistics.

In parts of Asia outside of the Middle East, drinking is not uncommon. South Koreans are the heaviest drinkers in Asia, according to the World Health Organization (WHO). It has been reported that South Koreans over the age of 15 on average drink

10.9 liters of alcohol a year. The country is famous for Soju, a fermented rice drink. Thailand came in second and Vietnam rounded out the top three when it came to the most alcohol consumers. Nearby Cambodia and The Philippines also had a large population of drinkers that is currently growing in numbers.

According to WHO, alcohol consumption in China is increasing faster than other parts of the world. One reason for the rise in drinking there is the country's fast economic development, giving way to higher income levels. It is sad to note that unlike the United States, the Chinese population has, for the most part, not caught on to the many dangerous myths concerning alcohol. Millions in China believe that alcohol relieves stress, which as you read earlier in this book, this is far from the truth. A recent national survey of drinking in China revealed that over 55% of the men and 15% of the women regularly consume alcohol. Just like in every other country where drinking is on the rise, more and more alcohol-related diseases are now being reported, and more horrifying drunk driving cases are taking place.

Across the sea from China, Japan is experiencing an alcohol crisis of its own. Unlike most of the industrial world, where drinking is decreasing, it is on the rise in the "Land of the Rising Sun." Alcohol plays a role in everyday life there, where young adults partake in two hour all-you-can-drink sessions and where it can be purchased from convenience stores 24 hours a day. It is estimated that over one million people suffered from Alcohol Use Disorder in 2013, which is 300,000 more than a decade earlier. However, only a fraction of them currently undergoing treatment. Just 40,000 to 50,000 are currently seeking help.

Unlike the United States, where celebrities often talk openly about their battles with Alcohol Use Disorder, it is difficult to find high-profile people in Japan who are willing to do the same. Only a very small handful have done so due to the fact that being dependent on alcohol is still viewed as a trait to be embarrassed about throughout that country. One of the few exceptions was the late Prince Tomohito of Mikasa, who was fifth in line for the throne before his passing in 2012. He spoke out about his drinking five years earlier in 2007. "The Imperial Household Agency had told me not to say outright that I am dependent (on alcohol) but I hated being made a topic of talk based on speculation," he once said on his decision to go public.

Dr. Susumu Higuchi reported in a 2014 *Japan Times* article that "Japan is a society that loves to push people to drink a lot. However, once someone becomes an addict, he or she is looked down on and it is not easy for that person to regain his or her status back in society after recovery." Unfortunately, Japanese lawmakers have been slow to address their country's drinking problem.

South of Japan, in Australia, alcohol dependency is frighteningly high among the population. The vast majority of citizens are worried that their drinking habits have become excessive. In a survey of over 1,800 people, 44% of Australians reported that they drink to get drunk and 35% claimed to have been affected by alcohol-related violence. In a country with a population of only 25 million people, the toll drinking has taken is shocking.

Every year there are 5,500 deaths in Australia that are the result of consuming this toxic liquid, along with 160,000 hospitalizations and 70,000 assaults. According to an online article produced by the *British Broadcasting Corporation*, "The World Health Organization ranks Australia 19th on the global alcohol consumption ladder, ahead of Ireland at 21, the UK at 25, New Zealand at 31, Canada at 40 and the United States at 48."

Alcohol is the second leading preventable cause of death and hospitalization in Australia after tobacco. Using different methods, the country is trying to combat its drinking issue. The government formed a program called Tackling Binge Drinking which attempts to promote a healthy approach to alcohol use, and also brings attention to the risk associated with alcohol. The nonprofit sector is also doing its share to help, with the organization Drink Wise, which provides information on handling teen drinking, binge drinking and drunk driving.

Over 14,000 away from "The Land Down Under," Europe is dealing with a severe crisis when it comes to alcohol use, especially in the nations that once made up the Soviet Union. The numbers of alcohol-related deaths are staggering in this region, with the life expectancies in many of these countries being shockingly low compared to the rest of the world.

As mentioned earlier, Russia is the nation with the world's worst drinking problems. Its population is the highest on the planet with those who suffer from Alcohol Use Disorder. This vast nation, the world's largest, stretches across two continents (Europe and Asia) and people who excessively abuse alcohol can be found in every city and town. Male life expectancy is only

64.3 years, significantly lower than other parts of the continent, due in part to alcohol-related issues. It was reported that in 2012, more than 30% of all deaths were the result of drinking.

The good news is Russians are actually starting to take a serious approach to reducing alcohol consumption in their country. While the life expectancy for men is low compared to elsewhere in Europe, it has actually risen from the years following the collapse of the Soviet Union in 1991. Just 25 years ago, the Russian male population had a 57.7 life expectancy rate.

Russian President Vladimir Putin has enacted new measures to restrict alcohol sales and to discourage use, such as increased taxation. In December of 2018 Russia's health ministry announced it was drafting legislation that could raise the country's drinking age from 18 to 21. Perhaps due to the fact that Russians are now starting to take their drinking issues seriously for what is likely the first time in its history, *The Moscow Times* cited a poll suggesting strong public support for the higher drinking age.

In the Scandinavian countries of Northern Europe, excessive drinking is a known problem. Cold and dark for most of the year, the citizens of these countries are prone to Seasonal Affective Disorder (SAD). Perhaps unaware, or simply not caring, about the fact that alcohol is a depressant, millions in this region drink in a desperate attempt to uplift their spirits, when in fact the alcohol use is doing the exact opposite. In Finland, alcohol is the number one killer of men, yet despite this, the government is loosening its alcohol policies.

In the case of Denmark, some may be surprised to learn there is no legal drinking age. There are only age limits when it comes to purchasing alcohol. At 16, Danes can start buying alcohol without any problem, and at 18 they are allowed to be served in bars and restaurants.

Unlike Denmark, Sweden has passed strict alcohol legislation, and purchasing drinks can be harder than many who reside outside the country might expect. The legal drinking age in Sweden is 20, and grocery and convenience stores are banned from selling anything other than beer below 3.5% strength. Systembolaget is a government-owned chain of liquor stores found throughout the country, however it is only open for short periods during the week. Monday through Wednesday, doors open at 10 am, but close at the strike of 6 in the evening, usually with a guard on hand to make sure every customer is out the door. Thursday and Fridays, it stays open only one hour later, closes at 3 in the afternoon on Saturdays and does not welcome buyers at all on Sundays. Not surprisingly, only 3.5% of deaths in Sweden can be contributed to alcohol. Drinking related deaths next door in Norway are also relatively low, with the regulations similar to Sweden's.

In Western Europe, drinking appears to be on the decline, with nations once famous for its wines (France) and beers (Ireland) seeing a drop in sales. Just like in the United States, more and more in this region are becoming more aware of the dangers alcohol poses. According to a 2018 *Irish Examiner* article, the World Health Organization reported alcohol consumption in Ireland has dramatically fallen by 25 percent since 2005. Alcohol use has also dropped in Southern Europe, including Italy, known for its wine tours. Over the last decade alcohol sales have decreased by 23 percent in that country.

While some nations in the Eastern Hemisphere continue to struggle with millions of people suffering from Alcohol Use Disorder, the good news is even hard drinking countries like Russia are becoming more aware of the damage this toxic liquid can have. Overall, drinking is down across the world. "Since 2000, the number of drinkers in the world has decreased by almost 5 percentage points, from 47.6 to 43.0, according to WHO," states a report from an October 2018 edition of *The Christian Science Monitor*. We can hope that this positive trend continues.

CHAPTER 8

Drinking Through History

Alcohol consumption is prevalent in today's world. As you have read in this book, drinking plays a significant role in the daily lives of countless people all over the globe. Today, in the 21st Century, alcohol is seen as a necessity. It is a celebrated, yet addictive, liquid that many cannot image life without. It is seen as an essential object to have on hand when we are celebrating an achievement, going out to dinner with an old friend, when we break up with a longtime partner and when we want to relax after a long day at work.

Why is that? Why do thousands of people across the planet feel like they need alcohol in order to function, in order to go about with life? To understand how we got to this point, we have to learn where we came from. We need to comprehend how alcohol has played a role in human history from its earliest recordings, and how we can move forward without it dominating the lives of so many people.

It is up to much debate how long humans as we are today have walked the earth. The estimate varies considering the source, and on what the exact definition of "modern man" entails. Using anthropology and science, we can narrow down the time when our ancestors first discovered alcohol and, how once it appeared, it grew in popularity to the extent that it would never fade away from human consumption.

It is likely that our ancient ancestors first happened upon alcohol in the form of fermented fruit by accident. At the University of Pennsylvania Museum in Philadelphia, Adjunct Professor Patrick McGovern is the Scientific Director of Biomolecular Archaeology Laboratory for Cuisine, Fermented Beverages, and Health. McGovern believes that once mankind became familiar with the intoxicating effect, they continued to pursue it.

As humans continued to evolve, so did the making of alcoholic beverages. When researching for this book, I found the history concerning the discovery of beer, liquor and wine to be extraordinarily fascinating. Equally intriguing is how these liquids, that have come to cause so much damage to countless people throughout history, have never disappeared from the human diet. Despite the devastating effect alcohol has on people, consumption has never decreased. Instead, it has grown to reach all corners of the globe.

It may never be known when beer was first discovered, however we do know that it developed in lands suitable for farming, and where there was enough time for grain fermentation. Around 5,000 years ago, it is believed that beer started to make its appearance in what was then Babylon, a kingdom in Mesopotamia (modern day Iraq). The ancient

Egyptians began brewing in the city of Hierakonpolis, located along the famous Nile River. It has been discovered that breweries in that particular city were capable of producing up to three hundred gallons of beer per day. Interestingly, however, numerous accounts of the period stressed the importance of drinking in moderation. And in 2018, one of the world's oldest breweries was found in a cave in Israel.

The discovery of beer was not limited to the Middle East, however, as there is evidence that it began to appear thousands of years ago in other continents as well. Evidence of beer making exist in what was once Pre-Columbian America. In 2007, the website *LiveScience* published an online article which stated that "Ancient Pueblo Indians brewed their own brand of corn beer, a new study suggests, contradicting claims that the group remained dry until their first meeting with the Europeans."

Wine also started to emerge on the scene more than a Millennia ago. According to a 2017 online article published by *National Geographic*, it is believed that chemical analysis now proves the Chinese used rice, honey and fruit to create wine just under 10,000 years ago. A few thousand years later, in what is now the nation of Georgia, wine started to gain popularity with people residing in the Caucasus Mountains. By domesticating grapes, mankind was able to produce the intoxicating beverage for those existing in this region. By the time of the ancient Greeks, wine was being produced on a household and communal basis, and was favored in Italy under the Roman Empire.

The taste for wine continued to grow, and in more recent centuries, its popularity started expanding into regions all over the world. During the 1700's, Europeans produced the addictive liquid in far off Australia. It was Governor Arthur Phillip who was responsible for bringing vines with him to the then largely unknown territory, which in turn created numerous vineyards in what is now present-day Sydney. Two centuries later, Australia started to become known worldwide for its wines. Today, people travel from all over the globe to experience wine tours in this South Pacific nation.

The history of liquor is equally fascinating. Just like beer, those who resided in ancient Babylon and Mesopotamia may have been some of the first to taste this intoxicating liquid. Today, certain liquors are associated with specific countries. For example, it is common knowledge that Mexico is known for its tequila, which is made from a blue agave plant that surrounds the city that bears the same name. In Russia, vodka reigns supreme. For hundreds of years, the people who populate this region have distilled the liquid from potatoes that have been fermented. However, some 21st Century brands use fruits or sugars instead.

Grapes, plants, potatoes; it doesn't sound like alcohol is harmful. However, nothing could be further from the truth. As stated earlier in this book, alcohol is ethanol. A 2017 *BBC* report summed it up perfectly when it stated, "Ripe fruits ferment and decay because of yeast that grows inside and on the fruits. Yeast breaks down sugar into alcohol, primarily ethanol – the alcohol in beer and wine." Ethanol is a toxic substance, as I explained in Chapter 4 titled *Alcohol And Our Health*.

Despite being a poisonous liquid, mankind has never stopped drinking. Why? The answer is simple: because it is addictive.

Alcohol has had a negative impact on people and nations for thousands of years, even altering the course of history. In 1223, the Russian Empire suffered a major blow – because of alcohol. That year, Mongol forces under the notorious ruler Genghis Khan, easily annihilated an enormous Russian army because the Russians had charged the battlefield while intoxicated. As a result, the Russian royalty was seized, and the Mongols expanded their borders.

As the centuries passed, man's addiction to this toxic liquid continued to grow. By the time the British started to settle the American Colonies in the 17th Century, drinking was becoming a daily routine. For nearly a year, "Spirited Republic: Alcohol in American History" was a popular exhibition at the National Archives in Washington D.C. Senior Curator Bruce Bustard remarked, "One of the things we understand now is that the initial ship that came over from England to Massachusetts Bay actually carried more beer than water." According to an interesting 2015 *BBC* report, "Early Americans even took a healthful dram for breakfast, whiskey was a typical lunchtime tipple, ale accompanied supper and the day ended with a nightcap. Continuous imbibing clearly built up a tolerance as most Americans in 1790 consumed an average 5.8 gallons of pure alcohol a year."

As the new nation formed and expanded west, alcohol consumption only increased. By the 19th Century, it peaked at a staggering 7.1 gallons a year, which in turn made it become a moral issue. Drinking was starting to have a serious impact on communities. As a result, the US Navy ended its long tradition of supplying sailors with a daily rum ration and talks of making alcohol straight out illegal started to grow throughout the country.

By the dawn of the 20th Century, support for Prohibition grew, making it a reality when the 18th Amendment was ratified on January 16, 1919. However, it is important to note that it did not prohibit the consumption of alcohol, but rather simply the sale, manufacture, and transportation of alcoholic beverages. Americans could not bring themselves to break their ties to drinking altogether, making way for the famous speakeasies of the 1920's. It wouldn't be until Americans were deep into the Depression that Prohibition ended. The 21st Amendment was passed in 1933, and alcohol was once again allowed to be sold throughout the nation.

Around the time Prohibition had started to gain traction in the United States, a man named Bill Wilson, who has come to be known to millions as "Bill W," was drinking his way through Europe. Born in Vermont in the fall of 1895, Wilson came from a long line of people who suffered from Alcohol Use Disorder. Perhaps surprisingly, he did not take his first sip of alcohol until his adult years, despite having been a child who routinely found himself in trouble at home and in school.

When World War I broke out in 1914, Wilson eventually joined the Allied Forces. It was during military training when he had his first drink, which was a glass of beer. It did not leave much of an impression on him. However, not long after he attended a dinner party in which he consumed cocktails for the first time. This time he enjoyed the toxic liquid, stating "I had found the elixir of life."

It wouldn't be long before he was thoroughly abusing alcohol, ruining much of his life in the process.

By 1935, Wilson realized he had to stop drinking or else he would likely die from it. He co-founded what is now known as Alcoholics Anonymous (AA) in Akron, Ohio. During this time, alcohol use disorder was commonly viewed as a moral failing. Back then, those in the medical field treated it as a condition that was not only likely incurable, but also lethal.

Drinking caused Wilson to lose just about everything good in his life. He never received his law degree because he was too drunk to pick up his diploma, and he couldn't maintain a successful career due to the fact he wouldn't quit consuming alcohol. Just before Wilson helped to form AA, he admitted himself to the Charles B. Towns Hospital for Drug and Alcohol Addictions in New York City under the care of Dr. William D. Silkworth. It was Silkworth's belief that alcoholism was a matter of both physical and mental control; that some had an inability to stop drinking once they started. This theory sat well with Wilson.

In the decades since its founding, AA has helped thousands of people all over the world gain back their sobriety. I applaud it for those it has helped. However, the reality is AA and the 12-Step program is nearly a century old. Even the term "alcoholic" is outdated and no longer recognized by most professionals in the addiction field. This is why I use the term "Alcohol Use Disorder" throughout this book, and why I rarely use the words "alcoholic" or "alcoholism."

Despite helping thousands of people win back their sobriety, AA has let thousands of others down. I am one of those people.

I gained absolutely nothing from sitting in a room and listening to someone else's story of addiction. Hearing these stories on a daily basis did not make me want to stop drinking, instead I found them so depressing that thoughts of "I wish I could go have a drink now" would flash through my mind. Watching people in these meetings become visibly upset because they were struggling with the desire to consume this addictive substance did not help my sobriety in any way. Equally unhelpful was the Alcoholics Anonymous "bible," *The Big Book.*

Having always been intrigued by history, I enjoyed portions of *The Big Book* in which Wilson talked about his life and adventures during and after World War I. However, once other people were introduced into the book, I lost interest. The book didn't seem to "flow" for me, and I was puzzled over why it was revered so much. Just like AA meetings, reading about people abusing alcohol did not aid my sobriety in any way, shape or form. Since gaining the courage to come forward and saying "Hey this whole AA thing didn't work for me. I found a different path," I have received emails and Facebook messages from grateful people all over the world who also have never gained much from those meetings and were thankful to learn that there are other ways to sobriety. You can't toss everyone into one box.

With all that being said, I certainly don't want to discourage anyone who enjoys AA from attending. If the program is working for certain people, then those individuals should certainly stick with it. However, for people like myself who find very little value in AA, there are other routes to sobriety, hence this book. This leads us to today, the 21st Century.

I wanted to go from feeling a desire to drink to no longer wanting to consume any alcohol. I didn't want to tell myself I couldn't drink, I wanted to tell myself I didn't WANT to do it anymore. That's when I saw the online advertisement for Annie Grace's book *This Naked Mind*. The timing was nothing short of a miracle, as I had all but come to terms with the fact that I would likely die from alcohol poisoning. I was prepared to become a statistic, as horribly sad as that thought is. However, when I read Grace's book, my entire outlook changed. Once I finished her incredible piece of work, the desire to drink was gone, and it literally happened overnight. It inspired me to write an article for her popular blog, which in turn lead me to publish this book.

As the 20th Century drew to a close, an alternative to AA emerged. Self-Management and Recovery Training (SMART) is a secular program that is rooted in science. Using cognitive behavioral therapy and non-confrontational motivational methods, it does not force people to admit they are powerless over addiction. Unlike AA, SMART does not embrace the theory that alcoholism is a disease. SMART Recovery believes that each individual finds his and her own path to recovery, which I applaud.

Today, in the 21st Century, huge scientific advancements are being made when it comes to overcoming addiction. At Scripps Ranch in San Diego, California, scientists have discovered how to reverse the desire to drink in alcohol-dependent rats. *Channel 10 News* in San Diego covered the story, in which it was reported that researchers were able to use lasers to inactivate a specific circuit in the brain to reverse the behavior. This is fascinating, encouraging news, and shows how far mankind has come when fighting addiction.

Throughout history mankind has been drawn to alcohol because of its addictive nature. It is a poisonous substance that has caused great armies to fall. As we continue to make our way through this new millennium, we are fortunate to live in a modern age in which we know the dangers of this toxic liquid. Unlike our ancestors who came before us, we are aware of the destruction it causes. It is our job to remember how alcohol has negatively impacted history, so history doesn't repeat itself. We owe it to the future generations.

Afterword

Once a person decides to cut back, or to quit drinking all together, he or she is often met with negative remarks by co-workers and friends. Most people who abuse alcohol know full well what they are doing, yet they live in a world of denial about the amount of drinks they consume. When those people consider changing their lifestyle to reduce the role alcohol plays in it, their peers become fearful. What do they fear? The thought of someone working to change his or her life for the better. Because deep down they are afraid that they cannot do the same. Therefore, they become defensive about their drinking, and try to discourage their friend from making the decision to quit.

Fortunately, I have not run into this. Every single person I know, from family members to friends to old high school teachers, have been extremely supportive of my decision to give up alcohol. However, I am unusually blessed in this department. Most people are not as lucky as I am. My friend Carlee, a single mother of a nine-year-old girl, is a perfect example of this.

A heavy drinker throughout her 20's and most of her 30's, Carlee knew she had a problem, but "normalized it" in her mind by spending time with what she referred to as her fellow "boozy mom" companions. They all drank, so she told herself it was okay, that what she was doing wasn't "that big of a deal." However, at the height of her drinking, Carlee was going through one, sometimes two, bottles of wine a night all on her own. When she finally decided that she wanted to change her lifestyle, her fellow drinking mothers were less than supportive. She sent me a copy of a text exchange she had with one of them. When Carlee wrote that she planned to stop consuming alcohol, the friend actually told her that quitting was "not realistic," and that she would not be able to fulfill her wish to change.

Thankfully Carlee realized that her friend's words were more of a reflection on herself, that the friend didn't want Carlee to stop because then she would have to admit she had a problem with drinking, too. When Carlee did quit, she sent me a text boasting about all the good in her life now that alcohol was no longer involved. She stated, "I've started a business and I hope to make a profit this year. I've noticed that I am so much more productive without alcohol."

Annie Grace sent out an email to her readers after she had published *This Naked Mind*. It went into detail about the treatment people who decide to quit drinking often receive from those who don't feel like they can limit their alcohol intake. The email stated: "Part of the fear of being a non-drinker with friends is that they think you won't be able to hang out anymore. I can still do everything I did before, but now the drink in my hand won't have alcohol in it. I can still let loose, have fun, dance all night and laugh until my stomach hurts. If the only tie that was binding us was alcohol, we probably weren't very good friends to begin with. My true friendships have not only continued as a non-drinker – they have improved."

Not having the support of your drinking peers or people you considered good friends is going to be something you will very likely encounter when you announce to them that you plan to cut back or quit drinking all together. Be prepared, and remember that most people experience this. Once they see you sticking to your decision to let go of alcohol and how well your life has improved because of it, they may be influenced by your strength and decide to cut back or completely eliminate drinking, too.

Carlee and Annie are not the only ones whose lives have greatly changed for the better since eliminating alcohol. While conducting research for this book, I came across countless positive stories from people all over the world who claimed that reducing their alcohol consumption, or quitting altogether, was the best decision they ever made.

One example is that of a woman by the name of Jennifer, who provided her story to a 2018 *Business Insider* article. Jennifer listed six reasons why giving up alcohol six years ago was the best decision she ever made, which included no longer suffering from hangovers, weeding out the not-so-great friends, spending more time with those she cares about the most, improving her chances of living a longer, healthier life, no longer embarrassing herself by being drunk, and saving money now that she isn't wasting it on drinks.

"Because I always opt for $2 Diet Cokes instead of $9 martinis when I go out, I have more cash in my wallet to save — or, let's be real, to spend on the late-night pizza that will call my name. Drinking is expensive. Sure, there are happy hour deals and well drinks if you're tight on money — but even those add up if you're out every weekend. I prefer to put my hard-earned dollars toward vacations or other experiences I'll actually be able to remember the next day," Jennifer stated.

Other people who completely eliminated alcohol from their daily lives did so because they saw it was taking them down a destructive path. Tim is one of those people. He provided his story to the website *Mind, Body and Green*, describing how his life improved drastically after just three weeks of leaving drinking in his past.

Like many people, Tim had spent his youth drinking with his friends and classmates. As he grew older, he leaned on alcohol to "solve" his problems. "Drinking worked to quell the loneliness and pulled me out of a few dark spots. In the long run, though, it perpetuated the issues I used it to escape from, and I knew if I kept up the way I'd been going, it would take a serious toll on my health. But I continued to cling to the idea that I could achieve my wildest professional dreams and live life to the fullest, while moderately and healthily drinking," he stated.

By the time he reached 30, one life altering event occurred that forced Tim to re-examine his dependency on alcohol. He got a DUI. Luckily no one was hurt, but it was the wake-up call he needed to put the bottle down for good.

"The fact that I had to make a choice was suddenly totally clear. I could stop drinking and keep evolving toward my highest self, or I could keep drinking and consciously limit myself and my achievements in this lifetime. When I saw it that way, it really wasn't a tough decision to make. Alcohol had to go." Tim continued, "Three weeks later, I haven't missed it one bit. I've been in liquor-laden environments, like dinner dates and rock concerts, and not experienced so much as a pang of longing. My fear that life wouldn't be as much fun has already transitioned into gratitude and appreciation for how present, clear, and focused I feel."

Like Jennifer, Tim listed additional examples of how no longer consuming this toxic liquid had greatly improved his existence, including one being an often-overlooked positive side effect: better skin! He stated that he no longer has "red blotches" on his face, and that it is now completely clear.

Tim's list also includes the fact that he no longer craves unhealthy "comfort" foods and is satisfied with more plant-based items, as well as having more energy during the day and no longer feeling the need for an afternoon nap. By eliminating alcohol, he has added yoga exercises and meditations to his daily routine, and his mind is much clearer. He stated, "I have much stronger focus, which means I get much more done. When I was drinking, there was no time for writing because my short-term memory was shot, and I spent my mornings recovering from the night before."

Perhaps most importantly Tim's social circle has changed for the better. He is now more interested in spending time with healthier individuals, claiming, "I can't think of a single reason to return to my former lifestyle. Try kicking your booze habit and see if you feel the same."

Deciding to ditch alcohol for good was also a smart move for Andy, a web developer from Chicago. He composed an article for the popular television show *Today's* website about his decision to ditch the drinking for good. Andy proudly informed a national audience, "I haven't slept this great since before high school. Man, it's fantastic. I could point you to all the studies that show how alcohol affects your sleep, but hey, take my word for it. This is the sleep I've dreamed of for years."

Andy mentioned that removing this toxic liquid from his life helped his mood, too. "I don't know if I have depression, but I used to get bummed out a lot. There were days when I wouldn't want to leave my apartment, or see anyone, mostly because I hated myself. I don't hate myself nearly as much as I used to. I'm generally OK with my life and who I am. Positivity is now my go-to emotion, even when something bad or terrible happens to me." He continued, "It's like I flipped this switch inside my brain: Instead of going to negativity, I try to find the reason something is positive. It's definitely weird to have this happen to me."

Andy ended by stating, "If you ever think, 'Hey, this drinking thing isn't fun anymore', it's fine to take a break. I just quit. For me, it's been relatively easy, and I know it isn't easy for everyone. But just know I've found countless rad people who can have fun without booze. And you can, too."

I can relate to how Annie, Carlee, Jennifer, Tim and Andy feel now that drinking no longer plays a role in my life. As I mentioned before, prior to when I started abusing alcohol, I was an extremely successful person for most of my life. I had some trials and tribulations during my teenage years that included battling Obsessive Compulsive Disorder, but I overcame that challenge better than anyone could have imagined. I even wrote a story about winning that battle, titled *Rediscovery*, which was published in two editions of the *New York Times* best-selling series *Chicken Soup for the Soul*.

I went on to college, where I made the Dean's List and wrote for the student newspaper. After receiving my B.A. in Communications, I went directly into graduate school, where I won a scholarship to study abroad at the prestigious Oxford University in the United Kingdom. After earning my M.A. in Public Policy, I spent several years working while enjoying life in different parts of the United States, from Washington D.C. to San Diego, California. During this time, I published two books on Russian History.

When the drinking took hold of me, I told myself I was self-medicating over the trauma that I touched on in the introduction of this book. While I was indeed using alcohol to numb the emotional pain, the truth is that during those successful years as a young adult, my tolerance to this toxic liquid had grown to a point I never would have dreamed of during my teenage and college years. That brief period of drinking uncontrollably nearly destroyed me. I am grateful it didn't steal too much time from my life; this only life that I have.

I am back to the person I use to be before the excessive alcohol use, but better. I am back to writing, traveling, and truly living life again. I enjoy the little pleasures once more, like the changing seasons and brilliant sunsets, but I have a newfound appreciation for them. I will never take another moment for granted, knowing how much alcohol almost cost me. I could have ended up like the homeless drinkers I see sitting on street benches every day, beer cans in their hands. I could have been too impaired to defend myself if a dangerous situation arose between myself and someone who wished me ill-will. Or I could have succumbed to alcohol poisoning, passing away on a cold bathroom floor, alone.

People sometimes ask me if I miss drinking, and the answer is a firm no. Many look at me, stunned. How could I not miss happy hours and summer cookouts with friends, they ask? The answer is I still attend social gatherings, I just drink a plain Diet Coke instead, and I'm perfectly happy with that. Think about it, if we gave up social gatherings, it wouldn't be the drinking we would miss, it would be the good company. I can still go to happy hours, summer cookouts, Christmas parties and other fun-filled events where there is drinking involved, I just don't consume any alcohol. I remind myself it isn't the toxic liquid I go for, it's the time spent with the people who make me laugh and brighten my day. Alcohol sure doesn't do that.

For most of my life, I've lived within a short drive of the beach, whether it be the Atlantic or Pacific Oceans. Many times, I would lay out on a large beach towel in the sand, watching the waves crash on the shore while sipping on a Margarita or some other mixed drink. I felt like I needed to do this in order to "truly enjoy" the beach experience. I now see how ridiculous that belief is. If I want a "beachy" drink on a hot summer day as I wade in the water, I can easily make a mixed drink, minus the alcohol. Just the other day I was enjoying the Florida sun and surf with a Pina Colada flavored energy drink, zero alcohol involved.

Guess what, the experience was just the same, if not better, than it would have been with an alcoholic beverage. Why better? Because I can actually remember the experience. The day's events aren't clouded by liquor.

If you are on the fence about taking your first sip of alcohol, I hope *Death In The Afternoon: How To Control Drinking In The 21st Century* has opened your eyes behind what is involved – and at stake – if and when you do start drinking. Down the road, if you start to question the amount of alcohol you are consuming on a regular basis, it is my sincerest wish that you refer back to this book as a guide to help you scale back – or quit entirely. If you already feel lost in your alcohol abuse, I hope this book helps to end your dependency on drinking and allows you to take your life back.

There is light at the end of what can seem like a very dark tunnel. I am living proof of it.

Made in the USA
Middletown, DE
30 October 2019

77553092R20057